YOUR GUIDE TO
Lowering Your Cholesterol With TLC

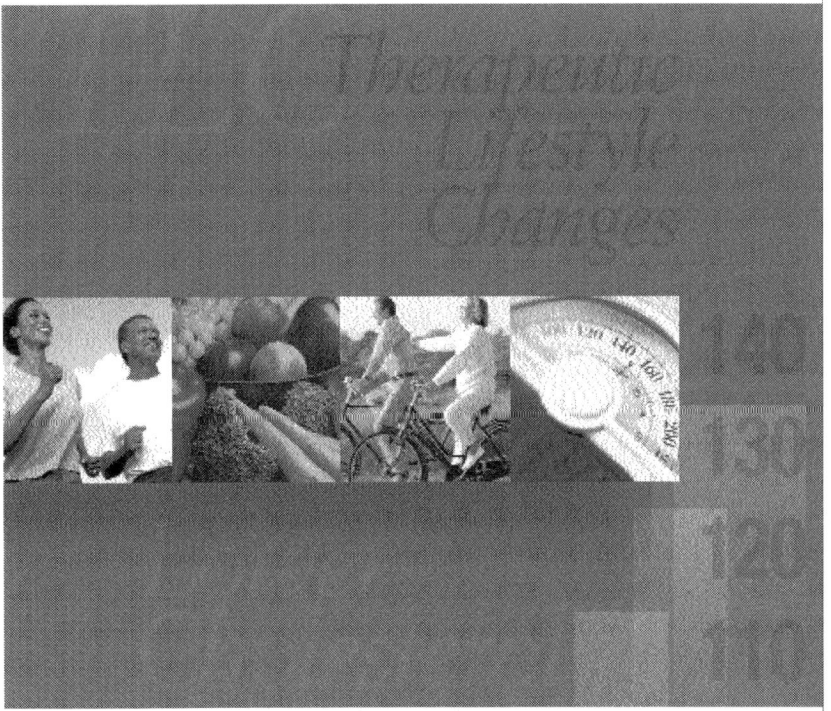

U.S. DEPARTMENT OF HEALTH AND HUMAN SERVICES
National Institutes of Health
National Heart, Lung, and Blood Institute

NIH Publication No. 06–5235
December 2005

Contents

Introduction 1

Why Cholesterol Matters 2
    What Affects Cholesterol Levels? 4
    Knowing Your Cholesterol Level 5
    Setting Your Goal 6

Treating High LDL Cholesterol 13
    The TLC Diet: A Heart Healthy Eating Plan 19
    Foods To Choose for TLC 30
    Becoming Physically Active 37
    Maintaining a Healthy Weight 43
    Sample Menus for TLC 54

The Metabolic Syndrome—A Special Concern 70

Learning to Live the TLC Way 73
    Keeping Track of Your Changes 73
    Be Smart When You Start 76
    Reward Yourself 76
    Making TLC a Family Affair 77

A Final Note 78

To Learn More 80

Introduction

High blood cholesterol can affect anyone. It's a serious condition that increases the risk for heart disease, the number one killer of Americans—women and men. The higher your blood cholesterol level, the greater your risk.

Fortunately, if you have high blood cholesterol, there are steps you can take to lower it and protect your health. This booklet will show you how to take action by following the "TLC Program" for reducing high blood cholesterol. TLC stands for Therapeutic Lifestyle Changes, a three-part program that uses diet, physical activity, and weight management. Sometimes, drug treatment also is needed to lower blood cholesterol enough. But even then, the TLC Program should be followed.

The booklet has four main sections: It explains why cholesterol matters and helps you find your heart disease risk; describes the TLC Program; talks about a condition called the metabolic syndrome that can also be treated with TLC; and offers advice on how to make heart healthy lifestyle changes. Within the sections you'll find tips on such topics as how to: communicate better with your doctor and other health care professionals, read food labels, make and stick with lifestyle changes, plan heart healthy menus for the whole family, and make heart healthy choices when you eat out.

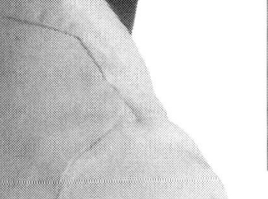

Anyone can develop high blood cholesterol—everyone can take steps to lower it.

Why Cholesterol Matters

Cholesterol is a waxy, fat-like substance found in the walls of cells in all parts of the body, from the nervous system to the liver to the heart. The body uses cholesterol to make hormones, bile acids, vitamin D, and other substances.

The body makes all the cholesterol it needs. Cholesterol circulates in the bloodstream but cannot travel by itself. As with oil and water, cholesterol (which is fatty) and blood (which is watery) do not mix. So cholesterol travels in packages called lipoproteins, which have fat (lipid) inside and protein outside.

Two main kinds of lipoproteins carry cholesterol in the blood:

- Low density lipoprotein, or LDL, which also is called the "bad" cholesterol because it carries cholesterol to tissues, including the arteries. Most of the cholesterol in the blood is the LDL form. The *higher the level of LDL* cholesterol in the blood, the greater your risk for heart disease.
- High density lipoprotein, or HDL, which also is called the "good" cholesterol because it takes cholesterol from tissues to the liver, which removes it from the body. A *low level of HDL* cholesterol increases your risk for heart disease.

If there is too much cholesterol in the blood, some of the excess can become trapped in artery walls. Over time, this builds up and is called plaque. The plaque can narrow vessels and make them less flexible, a condition called atherosclerosis or "hardening of the arteries."

This process can happen to blood vessels anywhere in the body, including those of the heart, which are called the coronary arteries. If the coronary arteries become partly blocked by plaque, then the blood may not be able to bring enough oxygen and nutrients to the heart muscle. This can cause chest pain, or angina. Some cholesterol-rich plaques are unstable—they have a thin covering and can burst, releasing cholesterol and fat into the bloodstream. The release can cause a blood clot to form over the plaque, blocking blood flow through the artery—and causing a heart attack.

When atherosclerosis affects the coronary arteries, the condition is called coronary heart disease or coronary artery disease. It is the main type of heart disease and this booklet will refer to it simply as heart disease.

Because high blood cholesterol affects the coronary arteries, it is a major risk factor for heart disease. Risk factors are causes and conditions that increase your chance of developing a disease. Other major heart disease risk factors are given in Box 1.

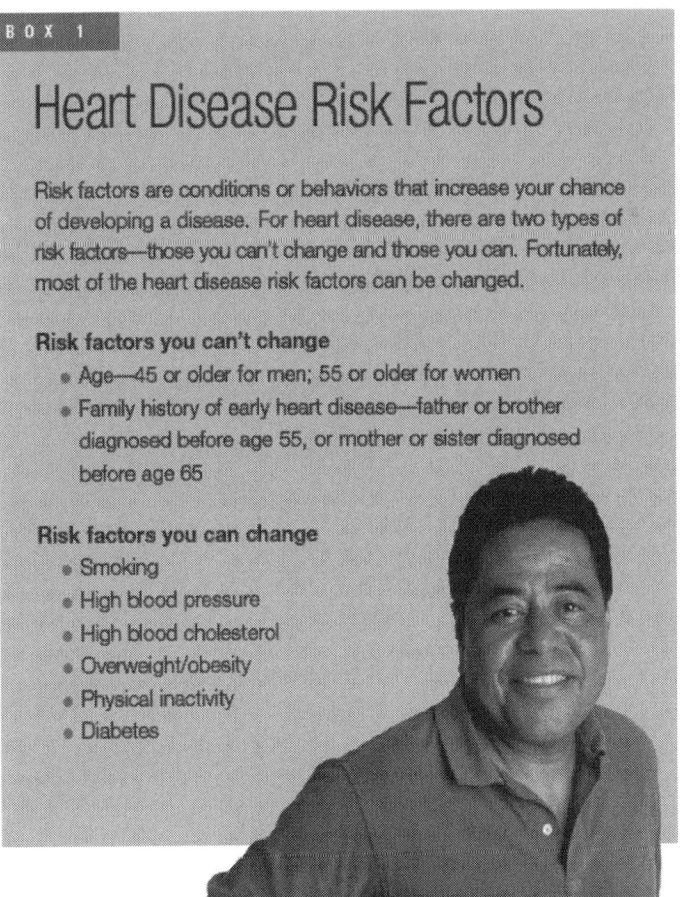

BOX 1

Heart Disease Risk Factors

Risk factors are conditions or behaviors that increase your chance of developing a disease. For heart disease, there are two types of risk factors—those you can't change and those you can. Fortunately, most of the heart disease risk factors can be changed.

Risk factors you can't change
- Age—45 or older for men; 55 or older for women
- Family history of early heart disease—father or brother diagnosed before age 55, or mother or sister diagnosed before age 65

Risk factors you can change
- Smoking
- High blood pressure
- High blood cholesterol
- Overweight/obesity
- Physical inactivity
- Diabetes

What Affects Cholesterol Levels?
Various factors can cause unhealthy cholesterol levels. Some of the factors cannot be changed but most can be modified. The factors are:

Those you cannot change—
- Heredity. The amount of LDL cholesterol your body makes and how fast it is removed from your body is determined partly by genes. High blood cholesterol can run in families. However, very few people are stuck with a high cholesterol just by heredity —and everyone can take action to lower their cholesterol. Furthermore, even if high cholesterol does not run in your family, you can still develop it. High cholesterol is a common condition among Americans, even young persons, and even those with no family history of it.
- Age and sex. Blood cholesterol begins to rise around age 20 and continues to go up until about age 60 or 65. Before age 50, men's total cholesterol levels tend to be higher than those of women of the same age—after age 50, the opposite happens. That's because with menopause, women's LDL levels often rise.

Those under your control—
- Diet. Three nutrients in your diet make LDL levels rise:
  - Saturated fat, a type of fat found mostly in foods that come from animals;
  - *Trans* fat, found mostly in foods made with hydrogenated oils and fats (see pages 20–21) such as stick margarine, crackers, and french fries; and
  - Cholesterol, which comes only from animal products.

  These nutrients will be discussed more later (see pages 19–23). But it's important to know that **saturated fat raises your LDL cholesterol level more than anything else in your diet.** Diets with too much saturated fat, *trans* fat, and cholesterol are the main cause for high levels of blood cholesterol—a leading contributor to the high rate of heart attacks among Americans.

- Overweight. Excess weight tends to increase your LDL level. Also, it typically raises triglycerides, a fatty substance in the blood and in food (see Box 2), and lowers HDL. Losing the extra pounds may help lower your LDL and triglycerides, while raising your HDL.

> **BOX 2**
>
> ## What Are Triglycerides?
>
> Triglycerides, which are produced in the liver, are another type of fat found in the blood and in food. Causes of raised triglycerides are overweight/obesity, physical inactivity, cigarette smoking, excess alcohol intake, and a diet very high in carbohydrates (60 percent of calories or higher). Recent research indicates that triglyceride levels that are borderline high (150–199 mg/dL) or high (200–499 mg/dL) may increase your risk for heart disease. (Levels of 500 mg/dL or more need to be lowered with medication to prevent the pancreas from becoming inflamed.) A triglyceride level of 150 mg/dL or higher also is one of the risk factors of the metabolic syndrome (see pages 70–72).
>
> To reduce blood triglyceride levels: control your weight, be physically active, don't smoke, limit alcohol intake, and limit simple sugars (see Box 20 on page 36) and sugar-sweetened beverages. Sometimes, medication also is needed.

- Physical inactivity. Being physically inactive contributes to overweight and can raise LDL and lower HDL. Regular physical activity can raise HDL and lower triglycerides, and can help you lose weight and, in that way, help lower your LDL.

Knowing Your Cholesterol Level

You can have high cholesterol and not realize it. Most of the 65 million Americans with high cholesterol have no symptoms. So it's important to have your blood cholesterol levels checked. **All adults age 20 and older should have their cholesterol levels checked at least once every 5 years.** If you have an elevated cholesterol, you'll need to have it tested more often. Talk with your doctor to find out how often is best for you.

The recommended cholesterol test is called a "lipoprotein profile." It measures the levels of total cholesterol (which includes the cholesterol in all lipoproteins), LDL, HDL, and triglycerides. The lipoprotein profile is done after a 9- to 12-hour fast. A small sample of blood is taken from your finger or arm. If you don't fast, you can still have your total cholesterol and HDL levels measured.

The levels are measured as milligrams of cholesterol per deciliter of blood, or mg/dL. Box 3 gives the classifications for total, LDL, and HDL cholesterol.

Setting Your Goal

The main goal in treating high cholesterol is to lower your LDL level. Studies have proven that lowering LDL can prevent heart attacks and reduce deaths from heart disease in both men and

---

BOX 3

Cholesterol Classifications

Total Cholesterol

Less than 200 mg/dL	Desirable
200–239 mg/dL	Borderline high
240 mg/dL and above	High

LDL Cholesterol

Less than 100 mg/dL	Optimal (ideal)
100–129 mg/dL	Near optimal/above optimal
130–159 mg/dL	Borderline high
160–189 mg/dL	High
190 mg/dL and above	Very high

HDL Cholesterol

Less than 40 mg/dL	Major heart disease risk factor
60 mg/dL and above	Gives some protection against heart disease

women. It can slow, stop, or even reverse the buildup of plaque. It also can lower the cholesterol content in unstable plaques, making them more stable and less likely to burst and cause a heart attack. Lowering LDL is especially important for those who already have heart disease or have had a heart attack—it will reduce the risk of another heart attack and can actually prolong life.

The level to which your LDL must be lowered depends on the risk for developing heart disease or having a heart attack that you are found to have at the start of treatment. The higher your risk, the lower your goal LDL level.

The TLC Program uses four categories of heart disease risk to set LDL goals and treatment steps. If you have heart disease or diabetes, then you are in category I, which has the highest risk. If you don't have either of those conditions, then find your risk category by doing the assessment in Box 4, which will send you to Box 5 if needed.

The higher your risk category, the more important it is to lower your LDL and control any other heart disease risk factors (including smoking and high blood pressure) you have. Further, the higher your risk category, the more you'll benefit from taking action. But whatever your risk category, you will use the TLC approach as a basic part of your treatment.

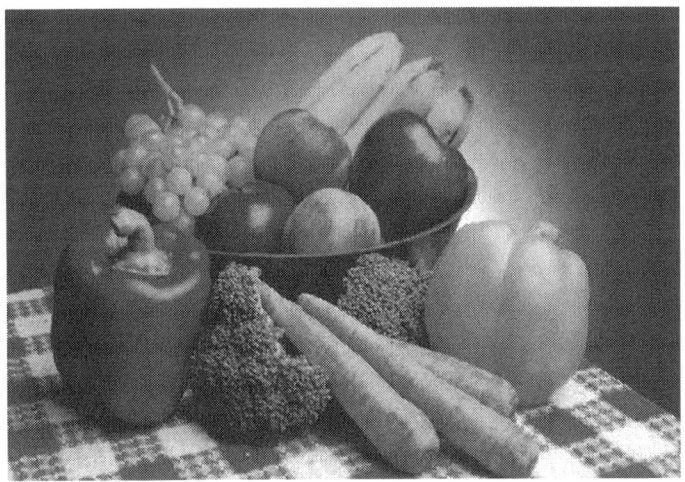

BOX 4

What's Your Heart Disease Risk?

Treatment for high cholesterol depends on your risk for heart disease. To find this risk and, so, your LDL treatment goal, answer the questions below—you may need to check with your doctor:

Step 1 How many of the following risk factors do you have? Check any that apply. Major risk factors that affect your LDL goal:

_____ a. Cigarette smoking
_____ b. High blood pressure (140/90 mmHg* or higher or being on blood pressure medication)
_____ c. Low HDL cholesterol (less than 40 mg/dL)†
_____ d. Family history of early heart disease (diagnosed in father or brother before age 55; diagnosed in mother or sister before age 65)
_____ e. Age (45 or older for men; 55 or older for women)

_____ Total number of risk factors (count the checks)

* mmHg stands for millimeters of mercury
† If your HDL is 60 mg/dL or higher, subtract 1 from your total count—that level gives you some protection against heart disease.

Note: Obesity and physical inactivity are not on the above list but must be corrected to keep your heart healthy. Diabetes is such a strong risk factor that by itself it gives you a high risk for heart disease (see Step 3).

Step 2 What is your risk of having a heart attack in the next 10 years? This is called a "risk score." If you have 2 or more of the risk factors in step 1, use Box 5 to get your risk score. If you have 0 or 1 of the factors in step 1, your risk score is low to moderate, and you can proceed to step 3.

Step 3 What is your heart disease risk category? Use your number of risk factors and your risk score to find your category in the table below.

Setting Your LDL Goal

Once you know your heart disease risk category, you can find your LDL goal level.

If you have:	You are in category:	Your LDL goal level is:
Heart disease, diabetes, or a risk score more than 20%	I—High Risk	Less than 100 mg/dL
2 or more risk factors and risk score 10–20%	II—Next Highest Risk	Less than 130 mg/dL
2 or more risk factors and risk score less than 10%	III—Moderate Risk	Less than 130 mg/dL
0 or 1 risk factor	IV—Low-to-Moderate Risk	Less than 160 mg/dL

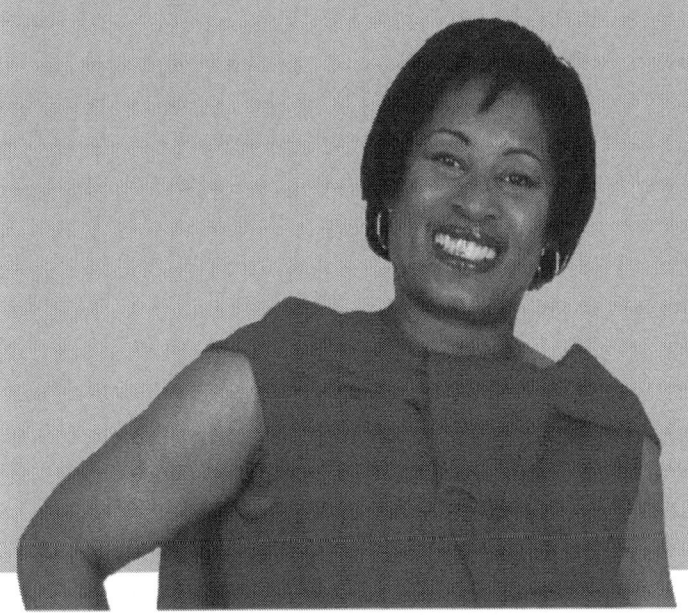

BOX 5

What's Your 10-Year Risk for a Heart Attack?

The tables below are based on data from the landmark Framingham Heart Study, a long-term study of the people in Framingham, MA, and their offspring. It gives you a risk score, or chance of having a heart attack in the next 10 years. Use the risk score to find your category of risk and your goal LDL level. A risk score of 20% means that 20 of 100 people in that risk category will have a heart attack within 10 years.

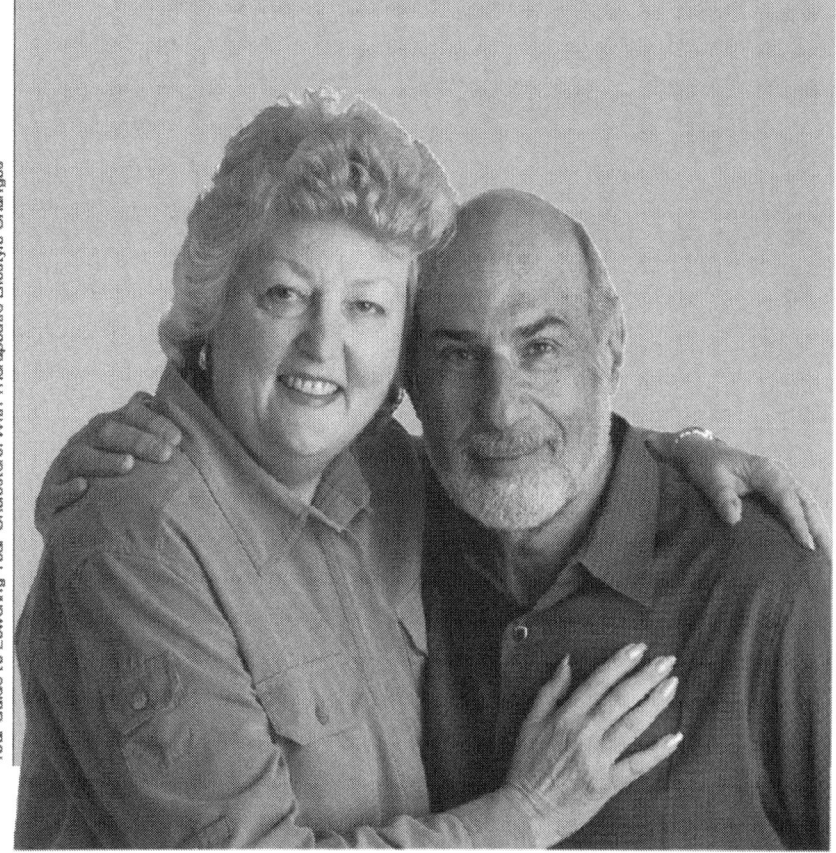

Estimate of 10-Year Risk for Men (Framingham Point Scores)

Age	Points
20–34	−9
35–39	−4
40–44	0
45–49	3
50–54	6
55–59	8
60–64	10
65–69	11
70–74	12
75–79	13

Total Cholesterol	Points				
	Age 20–39	Age 40–49	Age 50–59	Age 60–69	Age 70–79
<160	0	0	0	0	0
160–199	4	3	2	1	0
200–239	7	5	3	1	0
240–279	9	6	4	2	1
≥280	11	8	5	3	1

	Points				
	Age 20–39	Age 40–49	Age 50–59	Age 60–69	Age 70–79
Nonsmoker	0	0	0	0	0
Smoker	8	5	3	1	1

HDL (mg/dL)	Points
≥60	−1
50–59	0
40–49	1
<40	2

Systolic BP (mmHg)	If Untreated	If Treated
<120	0	0
120–129	0	1
130–139	1	2
140–159	1	2
≥160	2	3

Point Total	10-Year Risk %
<0	<1
0	1
1	1
2	1
3	1
4	1
5	2
6	2
7	3
8	4
9	5
10	6
11	8
12	10
13	12
14	16
15	20
16	25
≥17	≥30

10-Year risk _____ %

BOX 5 (continued)

Estimate of 10-Year Risk for Women (Framingham Point Scores)

Age	Points
20–34	-7
35–39	-3
40–44	0
45–49	3
50–54	6
55–59	8
60–64	10
65–69	12
70–74	14
75–79	16

	Points				
Total Cholesterol	Age 20–39	Age 40–49	Age 50–59	Age 60–69	Age 70–79
<160	0	0	0	0	0
160–199	4	3	2	1	1
200–239	8	6	4	2	1
240–279	11	8	5	3	2
≥280	13	10	7	4	2

	Points				
	Age 20–39	Age 40–49	Age 50–59	Age 60–69	Age 70–79
Nonsmoker	0	0	0	0	0
Smoker	9	7	4	2	1

HDL (mg/dL)	Points
≥60	-1
50–59	0
40–49	1
<40	2

Systolic BP (mmHg)	If Untreated	If Treated
<120	0	0
120–129	1	3
130–139	2	4
140–159	3	5
≥160	4	6

Point Total	10-Year Risk %
<9	<1
9	1
10	1
11	1
12	1
13	2
14	2
15	3
16	4
17	5
18	6
19	8
20	11
21	14
22	17
23	22
24	27
≥25	≥30

10-Year risk _____ %

Treating High LDL Cholesterol

Treatment for high LDL cholesterol involves the TLC Program and, if needed, drug therapy (see Box 6). But the cornerstone of your treatment is the TLC Program. Even if you need to take a cholesterol-lowering drug, following the program will assure that you take the lowest necessary dose. Further, the program does something drug therapy doesn't—it helps control other risk factors for heart disease too, such as high blood pressure, overweight/obesity, and diabetes, as well as the tendency of the blood to form clots.

As noted earlier, the TLC Program has three parts:

- Diet (see pages 19–41)
    - Decrease saturated fat, *trans* fat, and cholesterol.
    - Add plant stanols and sterols and increase soluble fiber.
- Physical activity (see pages 37–46)
- Weight management (see pages 43–57)

Box 7 (page 16) shows how much you can expect to lower your LDL cholesterol by following the TLC Program.

The intensity of your treatment will be tied to the degree of your heart disease risk. But whatever your degree of risk, you'll need to follow the TLC Program. This section gives you the steps to follow. The program uses a step-by-step approach to help make it easier for you to adopt the changes (see Box 8 on page 17). For instance, during the first 3 months of treatment, your main aim will be to lower your LDL cholesterol to its goal level through diet and physical activity. You will take in only enough calories to maintain a healthy weight, or achieve it if you're overweight.

You'll be working with your doctor and possibly other health professionals—see Box 9 (page 18) for tips on how to forge a heart healthy partnership. Your progress will be reviewed regularly and, if needed, your treatment will be adjusted to get your LDL cholesterol down to its goal level.

BOX 6

Cholesterol-Lowering Drugs

Many people will be able to lower their LDL enough with TLC alone. If your LDL needs more lowering, you may have to take a cholesterol-lowering drug in addition to TLC. However, by staying on the TLC Program, you'll be keeping that drug at the lowest possible dose, and as a bonus you'll be getting a bigger reduction in your risk for heart disease. So don't give up your heart healthy lifestyle changes.

There are various types of drugs used to lower LDL, and they work in different ways. Some may work for you, while others may not.

When you talk with your doctor about taking a cholesterol-lowering drug, be sure to mention other medicines you're taking—even over-the-counter remedies. And if you have any side effects from a medicine, tell your doctor as soon as possible. The amount or type of drug can be changed to reduce or stop bad side effects. If one drug does not lower your LDL enough, you may be given a second medication to go with it.

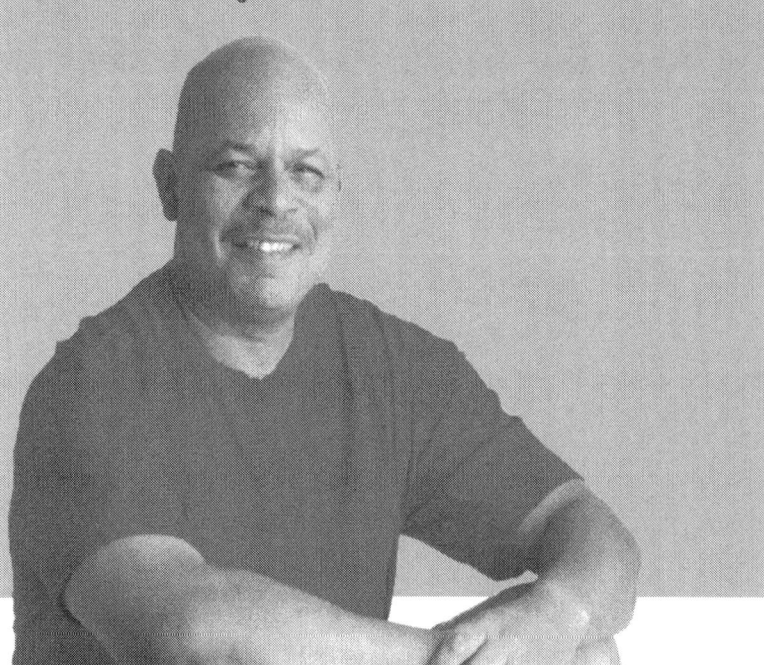

The major types of cholesterol-lowering drugs are:

- Statins—lovastatin, pravastatin, simvastatin, fluvastatin, atorvastatin, and rosuvastatin. Statins stop an enzyme that controls the rate at which the body produces cholesterol. They lower LDL levels more than other types of drugs—about 20–55 percent—and also moderately lower triglycerides and raise HDL.

- Ezetimibe. This drug reduces the amount of cholesterol absorbed by the body. Ezetimibe can be combined with a statin to get more lowering of LDL. Ezetimibe lowers LDL by about 18–25 percent.

- Bile acid resins. These bind with cholesterol-containing bile acids in the intestines and are then eliminated from the body in the stool. They lower LDL cholesterol by about 15–30 percent.

- Nicotinic acid—also called niacin. This is a water-soluble B vitamin that should be taken only under physician supervision. It improves all lipoproteins—total cholesterol, LDL, triglycerides, and HDL—when taken in doses well above the vitamin requirement. LDL levels are usually reduced by about 5–15 percent, and up to 25 percent in some patients.

- Fibrates. They mostly lower triglycerides and, to a lesser degree, raise HDL levels. Fibrates are less effective in lowering LDL levels.

Cholesterol-Lowering Drugs

BOX 7

Drop Your Cholesterol With TLC

You get a lot of benefit from the TLC Program. Here are some estimates of how much you can lower your LDL cholesterol by following various steps in the program. The estimates are what is expected based on research. The more you do with the program, the lower your LDL will go. Further, even if you take a cholesterol-lowering medication, you will still benefit from the program—it will keep the dose down.

	Change	LDL Reduction
Saturated fat	Decrease to less than 7% of calories	8–10%
Dietary cholesterol	Decrease to less than 200 mg/day	3–5%
Weight	Lose 10 pounds if overweight	5–8%
Soluble fiber	Add 5–10 grams/day	3–5%
Plant sterols/stanols	Add 2 grams/day	5–15%
Total		**20–30%***

*Notice that this amount of LDL reduction from TLC compares well with many of the cholesterol-lowering drugs.

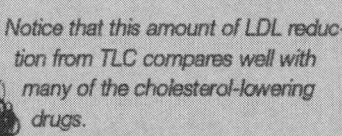

BOX 8

The TLC Path to Success

The TLC Program is a step-by-step way to lower your LDL cholesterol—and your heart disease risk. You'll start the program by following a heart healthy diet and becoming physically active, in addition to controlling other risk factors for heart disease such as smoking and high blood pressure. As you continue with the program, you and your doctor will review your progress toward reaching your LDL goal and, if needed, add other treatment options. Throughout the program, you may seek the advice of a dietitian or other health professional.

A typical TLC path to success would be:

First Doctor Visit—Start Lifestyle Changes
- Reduce saturated fat, *trans* fat, and cholesterol.
- Increase physical activity moderately.
- If overweight, reduce calories—increase fiber-rich foods to help reduce calorie intake.

—Allow 6 weeks—

Second Doctor Visit—Check LDL and, If Needed, Add More Dietary Approaches
- Reinforce reduction of saturated fat, *trans* fat, and cholesterol.
- Add plant stanols/sterols.
- Increase soluble fiber.

—Allow 6 weeks—

Third Doctor Visit—Check LDL and, If Needed, Add Drug Therapy
- Start drug therapy for LDL lowering, if needed.
- Focus on treatment of metabolic syndrome (see pages 70–72)—reinforce weight management and physical activity.

—Every 4 to 6 months—

Keep Checking Progress

BOX 9

Working With Your Doctor— A Healthy Partnership

Your doctor is your partner in treating your high cholesterol. The better you communicate with your doctor, the better you'll understand and carry out your treatment. This rule also applies to other health professionals who may join your treatment team, such as a dietitian or a physical activity specialist.

Here are some pointers on how to make your partnership work well:

- **Speak up.** If you don't understand something, ask questions. Even if you think you know the answer, ask and be sure you do. Ask for explanations in simple language.

- **Write it down.** Be sure you write down any treatment instructions. If you have trouble hearing, take a friend with you to the visit.

- **Keep records.** Record your test results at each visit.

- **Review your treatment.** Use your visit as a chance to go over your treatment plan. Check your goals. Be sure you're all in agreement over the next steps.

- **Be open.** If your doctor or another health professional asks you questions, give full and honest answers.

- **Tell if you're having trouble following the TLC Program.** Changes probably can be made so the program is easier for you to follow.

- **Tell any symptoms or side effects.** If something causes a side effect, briefly say what the symptom is, when it started, how often it happens, and if it's been getting worse.

The TLC Diet: A Heart Healthy Eating Plan

As noted earlier, what you eat greatly affects your blood cholesterol levels. That's why a key step in your treatment is to adopt a heart healthy eating plan—one that's low in saturated fat, *trans* fat, and cholesterol. Box 10 on the next page explains the different types of fat.

When you start on the TLC Program, you'll be asked to make dietary changes and to become physically active. The TLC diet calls for you to have:

- Less than 7 percent of your daily calories from saturated fat
- Less than 200 mg a day of cholesterol
- 25–35 percent of daily calories from total fat (includes saturated fat calories)
- Diet options you can use for more LDL lowering
  - 2 grams per day of plant stanols or sterols (see pages 27–28)
  - 10–25 grams per day of soluble fiber (see pages 23, 27–29)
- Only enough calories to reach or maintain a healthy weight
- In addition, you should get at least 30 minutes of a moderate-intensity physical activity, such as brisk walking, on most, and preferably all, days of the week.

More information about the nutrients of the TLC diet is given below. Throughout this booklet, you'll find tips on what foods to choose and how to prepare them, how to have healthy snacks, and how to dine out while staying on the TLC diet. The aim of the TLC diet is to help you eat healthier foods, cooked in healthier ways. This is not a temporary diet, but rather a new way of eating that is both heart healthy and tasty.

- **Saturated Fat** (see Box 10)

  As noted earlier, saturated fat raises your blood cholesterol more than anything else in your diet. That can't be stressed enough. You may read that *trans* fat raises cholesterol similarly to saturated fat, but it makes up far less of the American diet. The average person eats much more saturated fat than *trans* fat—about 4 to 5 times more. In fact, it's estimated that Americans eat an average of 11 percent of their total calories from saturated fat, compared with about 2.5 percent from *trans* fat.

> **BOX 10**
>
> ## The Skinny on Fats
>
> Fat is a nutrient that helps the body function in various ways: For example, it supplies the body with energy. It also helps other nutrients work. But the body needs only small amounts of fat, and too much of the saturated type will increase cholesterol in the blood.
>
> There are different types of fat, and they have different effects on cholesterol and heart disease risk. Here's a quick rundown (for more, see pages 19–23):
>
> - **Saturated fat.** This fat is usually solid at room and refrigerator temperatures. It is found in greatest amounts in foods from animals, such as fatty cuts of meat, poultry with the skin, whole-milk dairy products, and lard, as well as in some vegetable oils, including coconut and palm oils.
>
>   Studies show that too much saturated fat in the diet leads to higher LDL levels. Populations that tend to eat more saturated fat have higher cholesterol levels and more heart disease than those with lower intakes. Reducing the amount of saturated fat in your diet is a very effective way to lower LDL.
>
> - **Unsaturated fat.** This fat is usually liquid at room and refrigerator temperatures. Unsaturated fat occurs in vegetable oils, most nuts, olives, avocados, and fatty fish, such as salmon.

It's important to keep your saturated fat intake to less than 7 percent of your calories for the day—Box 11 on page 22 shows the grams of saturated fat you can have in a day for different calorie levels. Box 12 on pages 24–25 tells you how to use the food label to choose foods low in saturated fat.

■ *Trans Fat*

Trans fat—or *trans* fatty acids—is found mostly in foods that have been hydrogenated. Hydrogenation is a process in which

There are types of unsaturated fat—monounsaturated and polyunsaturated. When used instead of saturated fat, monounsaturated and polyunsaturated fats help lower blood cholesterol levels. Monounsaturated fat is found in greatest amounts in foods from plants, including olive, canola, sunflower, and peanut oils. Polyunsaturated fat is found in greatest amounts in foods from plants, including safflower, sunflower, corn, soybean, and cottonseed oils, and many kinds of nuts. A type of polyunsaturated fat is called omega-3 fatty acids, which are being studied to see if they help guard against heart disease. Good sources of omega-3 fatty acids are some fatty fish, such as salmon, tuna, and mackerel.

- **Trans fat.** Also called *trans* fatty acids, it tends to raise blood cholesterol similarly to saturated fat. *Trans* fat is found mainly in foods made with hydrogenated vegetable oils, such as many hard margarines and shortenings. The harder the margarine or shortening, the more likely it is to contain more *trans* fat.

- **Total fat.** This is the sum of saturated, *trans*, monounsaturated, and polyunsaturated fats in food. Foods have a varying mix of these types. The types of fat you eat have more to do with your LDL level than the total fat you take in—see above and pages 19–23.

hydrogen is added to unsaturated fat to make it more stable and solid at room temperature—and more saturated. Some *trans* fat also occurs naturally in animal fats, such as dairy products and some meats.

When you consume more unsaturated fat, you still must be careful to reduce your intake of *trans* fat. Main sources are stick margarine, baked products such as crackers, cookies, doughnuts, and breads, and foods fried in hydrogenated

> **BOX 11**
>
> ## Sample Saturated Fat Intakes
>
> In the war against an elevated blood cholesterol, your foremost foe is saturated fat. So the TLC Diet calls for you to have less than 7 percent of your daily calories from saturated fat. To help you follow that golden rule, here are some intakes for different daily calorie totals:
>
> | If you consume: | Eat no more than: |
> | --- | --- |
> | **Calories a day** | **Saturated Fat*** |
> | 1,200 | 8 grams |
> | 1,500 | 10 grams |
> | 1,800 | 12 grams |
> | 2,000 | 13 grams |
> | 2,500 | 17 grams |
>
> *Amounts shown are equal to about 6 percent of total calories.

shortening, such as french fries and chicken. *Trans* fat also may be in some unsuspected places, such as dietary supplements.

Soft margarines (tub and liquid) and vegetable oil spreads have lower amounts of *trans* fat than hard margarines. Some margarines are now free of *trans* fat.

A new Federal regulation requires the amount of *trans* fat in a product to be noted on the Nutrition Facts label of the food package by January 2006 (see Box 12 on pages 24–25). Use the label to choose margarines and other food products that have the least amount of saturated fat and *trans* fat. If *trans* fat is not listed on a product's Nutrition Facts label, check the ingredients list. Look for shortening or hydrogenated or partially hydrogenated vegetable oil—that often indicates the presence of *trans* fat.

Keep your intake of *trans* fat low. Be aware that *trans* fat is not included in the less than 7 percent of calories you can have from saturated fat.

- **Total Fat** (see Box 10 on pages 20 and 21)
  Not all fats raise cholesterol—that's why total fat is not itself a key target of your cholesterol-lowering treatment. But it's important to watch your total fat intake for a couple of reasons: Fat is calorie-dense and, if you need to lose weight, limiting your intake of it can help. Many foods high in total fat also are high in saturated fat. So eating foods low in total fat will help you eat less saturated fat. When you do eat fat, make it unsaturated fat—either monounsaturated (such as olive and canola oils) or polyunsaturated (such as safflower, sunflower, corn, and soybean oils).

  Total fat intake on the TLC Program can be from 25–35 percent of daily calories to allow flexibility in putting together a diet that works for you.

- **Cholesterol**
  The cholesterol in your diet raises the cholesterol level in your blood—but not as much as saturated fat. However, the two often are found in the same foods. So by limiting your intake of foods rich in saturated fat, you'll also help reduce your intake of cholesterol.

  Dietary cholesterol comes only from foods of animal origin, such as liver and other organ meats; egg yolks (but not the whites, which have no cholesterol); shrimp; and whole milk dairy products, including butter, cream, and cheese.

  Keep your dietary cholesterol to less than 200 milligrams a day. Use the Nutrition Facts label on food products to help you choose items low in cholesterol. See Boxes 12 and 13 (pages 24–26) for how to use food labels.

- **Soluble Fiber**
  Fiber comes from plants. Your body can't really digest it or absorb it into your bloodstream—your body isn't nourished by it. But it is vital for your good health.

  Foods high in fiber can help reduce your risk of heart disease. It's also good for your digestive tract and for overall health. Further, eating foods rich in fiber can help you feel full on fewer calories, which makes it a good food choice if you need to lose weight.

BOX 12

Read the Label

One of your best tools in working with the TLC diet is the Nutrition Facts label on the food package. It gives you the nutritional value and number of servings in an item.

You can use the label to compare foods and find ones lower in saturated fat, *trans* fat, total fat, cholesterol, and calories. First, you can compare and keep track of the actual number of grams of saturated fat, *trans* fat, or total fat, or the number of milligrams of cholesterol, or the number of calories in different foods. Second, you can use the Percent Daily Value listing for all but *trans* fat.* This tells you how much each serving of the item supplies of the day's recommended intake of various nutrients for people who do not have a cholesterol problem and whose diet therefore allows slightly more saturated fat and cholesterol than the TLC diet. Even though not all the percents shown are exactly right for TLC, you can still use them to compare foods. As a guide, if you want to consume less of a nutrient (such as saturated fat, cholesterol, or sodium), choose foods with a lower percent daily value—5 percent or less is low. If you want to consume more of a nutrient (such as fiber), seek foods with a higher Percent Daily Value—20 percent or more is high.

Also get in the habit of checking an item's ingredients list. It will tell you what the product contains—including any added nutrients, fats, or sugars. Ingredients are listed in descending order of amount by weight.

If you're trying to lose weight, pay particular attention to the number of servings per container. It's all too easy to mistake the calories per serving for the product's total calories.

See Box 13 for information on how to decipher the special content claims on food labels.

* The label will not show a Percent Daily Value for trans fat because a recommended daily intake has not been set for trans fat.

Light Margarine

Nutrition Facts

Serving Size 1 Tbsp (14g)
Servings Per Container 80

Amount Per Serving

Calories 50   Calories from Fat 50

% Daily Value*

Total Fat 6g	9%
Saturated Fat 1.5g	8%
Trans Fat 0g	
Cholesterol 0mg	2%
Sodium 55mg	2%
Total Carbohydrate 0g	0%
Dietary Fiber 0g	0%
Sugar 0g	
Protein 0g	

Vitamin A	10%	Calcium	0%
Vitamin E	8%	Iron	0%
Vitamin C	0%		

*Percent Daily Values are based on a 2,000 calorie diet. Your Daily Values may be higher or lower depending on your calorie needs.

	Calories	2,000	2,500
Total Fat	Less than	65g	80g
Sat. Fat	Less than	20g	25g
Cholesterol	Less than	300mg	300mg
Sodium	Less than	2,400mg	2,400mg
Total Carbohydrate		300g	375g
Dietary Fiber		25g	30g

Start here

Check calories

Limit these

Get enough of these

Quick guide to % Daily Value

- 5% or less is low
- 20% or more is high

Read the Label

BOX 13

Learn the Label Language

Food labels should be your new best friends. They'll help you find heart healthy products. Various terms are used—from "free" to "lean." Some terms are used interchangeably—"little," "few," and "low source of" are used to mean "low." Here is a translation of what some of the terms mean—look for these terms when choosing heart healthy items:

Phrase	What It Means
For Fats, Cholesterol, Sodium, and Meat:	
Fat free	Less than 0.5 grams per serving
Low saturated fat	1 gram or less per serving
Low fat	3 grams or less per serving
Reduced fat	At least 25 percent less fat per serving than the regular version
Light (in fat)	Half the fat of the regular version
Low cholesterol	20 milligrams or less per serving, and 2 grams or less of saturated fat per serving
Low sodium	140 milligrams or less per serving
Lean	Less than 10 grams of fat, 4.5 grams or less of saturated fat, and less than 95 milligrams of cholesterol per serving
Extra Lean	Less than 5 grams of fat, less than 2 grams of saturated fat, and less than 95 milligrams of cholesterol per serving
For Calories:	
Calorie free	Less than 5 calories per serving
Low calorie	40 calories or less per serving
Reduced or less calories	At least 25 percent fewer calories per serving than the regular version
Light or lite	Half the fat or a third of the calories of the regular version

There are two main types of fiber—insoluble and soluble (also called "viscous"). Both have health benefits but only soluble fiber reduces the risk of heart disease. It does that by helping to lower LDL cholesterol.

The difference between the two types is how they go through the digestive tract. Insoluble fiber goes through it largely undissolved. It's also called "roughage" and helps the colon function properly. It's found in many whole-grain foods, fruits (with the skins), vegetables, and legumes (such as dry beans and peas).

Soluble fiber dissolves into a gel-like substance in the intestines. The substance helps to block cholesterol and fats from being absorbed through the wall of the intestines into the blood stream. Research shows that people who increased their soluble fiber intake by 5–10 grams each day had about a 5 percent drop in their LDL cholesterol. TLC recommends that you get at least 5–10 grams of soluble fiber a day—and, preferably, 10–25 grams a day, which will lower your LDL even more.

Box 14 offers some easy ways to increase your intake of soluble fiber. Box 15 shows good sources of soluble fiber and gives you the amount of soluble and total fiber in those foods.

One caution: Increase the amount of fiber in your diet gradually, rather than all at once. A sudden increase in fiber can cause abdominal cramps or bloating.

■ Plant Stanols and Sterols

Plant stanols and sterols occur naturally in small amounts in many plants. Those used in food products are taken from soybean and tall pine-tree oils. When combined with a small amount of canola oil, the product is used in various foods.

As with soluble fiber, plant stanols and sterols help block the absorption of cholesterol from the digestive tract, which helps to lower LDL—without affecting HDL or triglycerides. Studies show that a daily intake of about 2 grams of either stanols or sterols reduces LDL cholesterol by about 5–15 percent—often within weeks.

> **BOX 14**
>
> ## Fiber Solutions
>
> How can you add soluble fiber to your diet? It's easy. Here are some quick tips:
>
> - Choose hot or cold breakfast cereals such as oatmeal and oatbran that have 3–4 grams of fiber per serving.
> - Add a banana, peach, apple, berries, or other fruit to your cereal.
> - Eat the whole fruit instead of, or in addition to, drinking its juice—one orange has six times more fiber than one 4-ounce glass of orange juice.
> - Add black, kidney, white, pinto, or other beans, or lentils to salads.

Stanols and sterols are added to certain margarines and some other foods, such as a special type of orange juice. But remember that foods with stanols/sterols are not calorie-free. If you use these products, you may need to offset the calories by cutting back elsewhere.

■ Other Dietary Factors

The following dietary factors may not affect LDL levels but you should be aware of their relationship to heart health:

Omega-3 Fatty Acids—Omega-3 fats are found in some fatty fish and in some plant sources, such as walnuts, canola and soybean oils, and flaxseed. They do not affect LDL levels but may help protect the heart in other ways. In some studies, people who ate fish had a reduced death rate from heart disease. It is possible that this is related to the effects of omega-3 fats, which may help prevent blood clots from forming and inflammation from affecting artery walls. Omega-3 fats also may reduce the risk for heart rhythm problems and, at high doses, reduce triglyceride levels. Studies have suggested that omega-3 fats reduce the risk for heart attack and death from heart disease for those who already have heart disease.

Based on what is now known, try to have about two fish meals every week. Fish high in omega-3 fats are salmon, tuna (even

BOX 15

Fiber Really Counts

Here are some soluble fiber and total fiber amounts (in grams) for various foods:

	Soluble	Total
Whole-grain cereals—½ cup cooked (except where noted)		
• Barley	1	4
• Oatmeal	1	2
• Oatbran	1	3
• Psyllium seeds, ground (1 Tbsp)	5	6
Fruit—1 medium (except where noted)		
• Apple	1	4
• Banana	1	3
• Blackberries (½ cup)	1	4
• Citrus (orange, grapefruit)	2	2–3
• Nectarine	1	2
• Peach	1	2
• Pear	2	4
• Plum	1	1.5
• Prunes (¼ cup)	1.5	3
Legumes—½ cup cooked		
• Black beans	2	5.5
• Kidney beans	3	6
• Lima beans	3.5	6.5
• Navy beans	2	6
• Northern beans	1.5	5.5
• Pinto beans	2	7
• Lentils (yellow, green, orange)	1	8
• Chick peas	1	6
• Black-eyed peas	1	5.5
Vegetables—½ cup cooked		
• Broccoli	1	1.5
• Brussels sprouts	3	4.5
• Carrots	1	2.5

canned), and mackerel. Pregnant women and nursing mothers should avoid some types of fish and eat types lower in mercury. See the Web site www.cfsan.fda.gov/~dms/admehg3.html for more information.

Sodium—Studies have found that reducing the amount of sodium in your diet lowers blood pressure. High blood pressure is a major risk factor for heart disease.

Sodium is one component of table salt (sodium chloride). But it's found in other forms too. So read food labels. Some low fat foods are high in sodium—use the label to choose the lower sodium options. Vegetables and fruits are naturally low in sodium—and low in saturated fat and calories. For more on salt, see Box 16.

Instead of using salt or added fat to make foods tastier, use spices and herbs. Box 17 on page 32 tells how to spice up meals.

- **Alcohol**—You may have heard that moderate drinking reduces the risk for heart disease. Small amounts of alcohol may help protect some persons.

However, drinking too much alcohol can have serious health consequences. It can damage the heart and liver, and contribute to both high blood pressure and high triglycerides.

If you don't drink now, don't start. If you do drink, have no more than one drink a day for women and two a day for men. Box 18 on page 33 gives some examples of what one drink equals.

And don't forget that alcohol has calories. If you need to lose weight, you will need to be especially careful about how many alcoholic beverages you drink.

Foods To Choose for TLC

The TLC diet encourages you to choose a variety of nutritious and tasty foods. Choose fruits, vegetables, whole grains, low-fat or non-fat dairy products, fish, poultry without the skin, and, in moderate amounts, lean meats. Box 19 (pages 34–35) shows the foods to choose and the number of servings by food group. Box 20 on page

BOX 16

A Word About Salt

Salt is sodium chloride. If you have high blood pressure, your doctor may tell you to cut down on salt and other forms of sodium.

All Americans should limit their sodium intake to no more than 2,300 milligrams of sodium (about 1 teaspoon of salt) a day—that includes all sodium consumed, whether added in cooking or at the table, or already present in food products. In fact, processed foods account for most of the salt and sodium Americans consume.

You may be surprised at which products have sodium. They include soy sauce, seasoned salts, monosodium glutamate (MSG), baking soda, and some antacids. Be sure to read food labels to choose products lower in sodium.

Fresh fruits and vegetables are naturally low in sodium. But canned fruits and vegetables

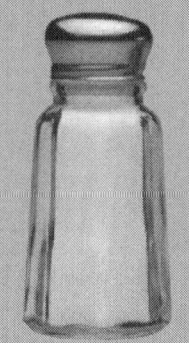

36 gives you information on carbohydrates in your diet, and information about fats is provided in Box 10 (pages 20–21).

A Word About Fruits and Vegetables

Eating more fruits and other low-fat foods is a good way to cut down on saturated fat. Fresh fruits offer great taste and variety—and, as a bonus, they require little or no preparation. Dried fruits can be carried with you, even in the car, and make a handy snack—try mixing raisins with nuts. One caution: If you're watching your calories, you may need to limit your intake of dried fruits and nuts. A serving of dried fruits is only ¼ cup.

BOX 17

Spice It Up!

Less salt? Less fat? Don't worry. You can make your mealtimes tasty by using spices and herbs. Here are some guidelines on what goes best with what:

For Meat, Poultry, and Fish

Beef	Bay leaf, marjoram, nutmeg, onion, pepper, sage, thyme
Lamb	Curry powder, garlic, rosemary, mint
Pork	Garlic, onion, sage, pepper, oregano
Veal	Bay leaf, curry powder, ginger, marjoram, oregano
Chicken	Ginger, marjoram, oregano, paprika, poultry seasoning, rosemary, sage, tarragon, thyme
Fish	Curry powder, dill, dry mustard, lemon juice, marjoram, paprika, pepper

For Vegetables

Carrots	Cinnamon, cloves, marjoram, nutmeg, rosemary, sage
Corn	Cumin, curry powder, onion, paprika, parsley
Green beans	Dill, curry powder, lemon juice, marjoram, oregano, tarragon, thyme
Greens	Onion, pepper
Peas	Ginger, marjoram, onion, parsley, sage
Potatoes	Dill, garlic, onion, paprika, parsley, sage
Summer squash	Cloves, curry powder, marjoram, nutmeg, rosemary, sage
Winter squash	Cinnamon, ginger, nutmeg, onion
Tomatoes	Basil, bay leaf, dill, marjoram, onion, oregano, parsley, pepper

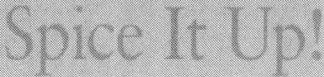

BOX 18

A Drink Equals

If you drink alcoholic beverages, do so in moderation. Women should have no more than one alcoholic drink a day and men no more than two. Here's what counts as one drink—along with the calorie content in case you need to lose weight:

- 12 ounces of beer—150 calories
- 5 ounces of wine—100 calories
- 1 ½ ounces of 80-proof hard liquor—100 calories

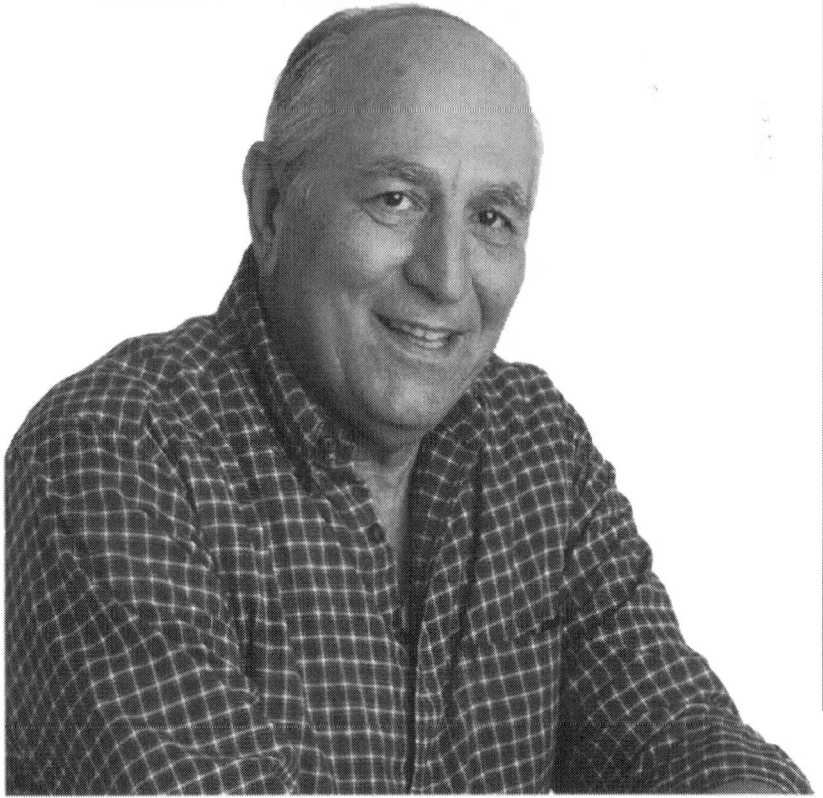

BOX 19

Eating Well With TLC

The TLC Diet calls for a variety of foods that are low in saturated fat, *trans* fat, and cholesterol but high in taste. It is not a deprivation diet. It can satisfy your taste buds as much as your heart. Here's the breakdown of the TLC diet by food groups (see Box 33 on page 55 for a guide to serving sizes):

Breads/Cereals/ Grains	**6 or more servings a day—adjust to calorie needs**
	Foods in this group are high in complex carbohydrates (see Box 20 on page 36) and fiber. They are usually low in saturated fat, cholesterol, and total fat.
	Whole-grain breads and cereals, pasta, rice, potatoes, low-fat crackers, and low-fat cookies
Vegetables/ Dry Beans/Peas	**3–5 servings a day**
	These are important sources of vitamins, fiber, and other nutrients. Dry beans/peas are fiber-rich and good sources of plant protein.
	Fresh, frozen, or canned—without added fat, sauce, or salt
Fruits	**2–4 servings a day**
	These are important sources of vitamins, fiber, and other nutrients.
	Fresh, frozen, canned, dried—without added sugar
Dairy Products	**2–3 servings a day—fat free or low fat (for example, 1% milk)**
	These foods provide as much or more calcium and protein than whole milk dairy products—but with little or no saturated fat.
	Fat-free or low-fat milk, buttermilk, yogurt, sour cream, cream cheese, low-fat cheese (with no more than 3 grams of fat per ounce, such as low-fat cottage cheese)
Eggs	**2 or fewer yolks per week—including yolks in baked goods and in cooked or processed foods.**
	Yolks are high in dietary cholesterol. Egg whites or egg substitutes have no cholesterol and less calories than whole eggs.

Meat/Poultry/Fish	**5 or less ounces a day**
	Poultry without skin and fish are lower in saturated fat. Lean cuts of meat have less fat and are rich sources of protein and iron. Be sure to trim any fat from meat and remove skin from poultry before cooking.
	Lean cuts of beef include sirloin tip, round steak, and rump roast; extra lean hamburger; cold cuts made with lean meat or soy protein; lean cuts of pork are center cut ham, loin chops, and pork tenderloin
	Strictly limit organ meats, such as brain, liver, and kidneys—they are high in cholesterol.
	Eat shrimp only occasionally—it is moderately high in cholesterol.
Fats/Oils	**Amount depends on daily calorie level**
	Nuts are high in calories and fat, but have mostly unsaturated fat. Nuts can be eaten in moderation on the TLC diet—be sure the amount you eat fits your calorie intake.
	Unsaturated vegetable oils that are high in unsaturated fat (such as canola, corn, olive, safflower, and soybean); soft or liquid margarines (the first ingredient on the food label should be unsaturated liquid vegetable oil, rather than hydrogenated or partially hydrogenated oil) and vegetable oil spreads; salad dressings; seeds; nuts.
	Choose products that are labeled "low-saturated fat," which equals 1 gram of saturated fat per serving.
Diet Options:	
Stanol/sterol–containing food products (see pages 27–28)	Specially labeled margarines and orange juice
Soluble fiber	Barley, oats, psyllium, apples, bananas, berries, citrus fruits, nectarines, peaches, pears, plums, prunes, broccoli, brussels sprouts, carrots, dry beans, peas, soy products (such as tofu, miso)

BOX 20

CARBS—Good, Bad, or What?

"Carbs," or carbohydrates, seem to be making a lot of news these days. Are they good or bad—in fact, what are they?

They're your body's main source of energy. They include fibers, starches, and sugars—in short, everything from bagels to rice to pineapples to lima beans. Even yogurt has carbohydrates. But they can be broken down into two main types—complex and simple.

Complex carbohydrates are just that—they have a more complex chemical structure than simple carbohydrates. Complex carbohydrates include starches and fiber. Examples are cereals, pastas, rice, vegetables, and fruits. Many are low in calories and high in fiber. They're a key part of a healthy eating plan.

Simple carbohydrates are sugars and include candy and other sweets. They tend to be high in calories and low in nutrients. So reducing the amount of simple sugars and sugar-containing beverages in your diet can help you cut down on calories and lose weight.

Some diets tout a "low carb" solution to weight gain. But the key to weight management is really calories, not which foods they come from. As with other sources of calories (fats and proteins), carbohydrates make you gain weight if you eat more calories than you use up.

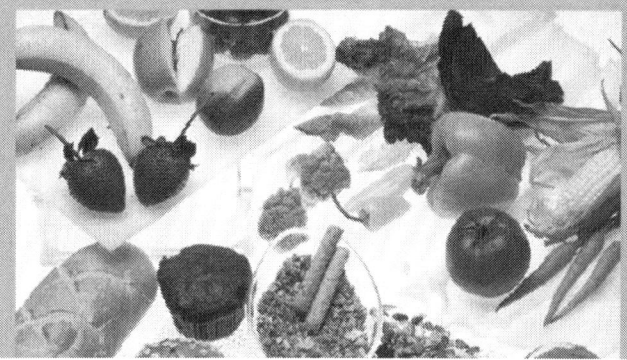

Eating more fruits and vegetables has another benefit too: It will make your diet richer in fiber, vitamins (such as the antioxidants C, E, and beta-carotene), and minerals. As a further plus, fresh fruits and vegetables are low in sodium.

What About Dessert?
The TLC diet lets you have moderate amounts of sweets and low-saturated fat desserts. Box 21 offers some suggestions for healthy snacks and desserts.

Cooking With TLC
It's not just what you eat but how you prepare food that matters. Box 22 (pages 39–40) offers advice on cooking methods to keep meals low in saturated fat. The box also gives tips on how to make recipes healthier.

Eating Out With TLC
You can eat out in restaurants and go to parties while on the TLC diet. Box 23 (page 41) gives you some tips for staying on TLC at restaurants and social events.

Becoming Physically Active
Becoming physically active is another key part of the TLC Program —it's a step that has many benefits.

Lack of physical activity is a major risk factor for heart disease. It affects your risk of heart disease both on its own and by its effects on other major risk factors. Regular physical activity can help you manage your weight and, in that way, help lower your LDL. It also can help raise HDL and lower triglycerides, improve the fitness of your heart and lungs, and lower blood pressure. And it can reduce your risk for developing diabetes or, if you already have the condition, lessen your need for insulin. Other benefits of regular physical activity are listed in Box 24 (page 42).

You don't have to run marathons to become physically active. In fact, if you haven't been active, the key to success is starting slowly and gradually increasing your effort. For instance, start by taking a walk during breaks at work and gradually lengthen your walks or increase your pace.

If you have heart disease or high blood pressure, or if you are a man over 40 or a woman over 50 who is planning to be very active, you

BOX 21

TLC Snacks and Treats

Eating the TLC way doesn't mean depriving yourself of snacks and treats. Try these low-saturated fat munchies and desserts—*but keep track of the calories:*

Snacks
- Fresh or frozen fruits
- Fresh vegetables
- Pretzels
- Popcorn (air popped or cooked in small amounts of vegetable oil and without added butter or salt)
- Low-fat or fat-free crackers (such as animal crackers, fig and other fruit bars, ginger snaps, and molasses cookies)
- Graham crackers
- Rye crisp
- Melba toast
- Bread sticks
- Bagels
- English muffins
- Ready-to-eat cereals

Desserts and sweets
- Fresh or frozen fruits
- Low-fat or fat-free fruit yogurt
- Frozen low-fat or fat-free yogurt
- Low-fat ice cream
- Fruit ices
- Sherbet
- Angel food cake
- Jello
- Baked goods, such as cookies, cakes, and pies with pie crusts, made with unsaturated oil or soft margarines, egg whites or egg substitutes, and fat-free milk
- Candies with little or no fat, such as hard candy, gumdrops, jelly beans, and candy corn

BOX 22

How to Make Heart Healthy Meals

Eating heart healthy meals doesn't mean giving up on taste. Here are some tips on how to make "health" a special ingredient in your recipes:

Cooking Methods
- Use low-fat methods and remember not to add butter or high-fat sauces—Bake, broil, microwave, roast, steam, poach, lightly stir fry or sauté in cooking spray, small amount of vegetable oil, or reduced sodium broth, grill seafood, chicken, or vegetables.
- Use a nonstick (without added fat) or regular (with small amount of fat) pan.
- Chill soups and stews for several hours and remove congealed fat.
- Limit salt in preparing stews, soups, and other dishes—use spices and herbs to make dishes tasty.

Milk/Cream/Sour Cream
- Cook with low-fat (1-percent fat) or fat-free types of milk or of evaporated milk, instead of whole milk or cream.
- Instead of sour cream, blend 1 cup low-fat, unsalted cottage cheese with 1 tablespoon fat-free milk and 2 tablespoons lemon juice, or substitute fat-free or low-fat sour cream or yogurt.

Spices/Flavorings
- Use a variety of herbs and spices in place of salt (see Box 17 on page 32).
- Use low-sodium bouillon and broths, instead of regular bouillons and broths.
- Use a small amount of skinless smoked turkey breast instead of fatback to lower fat content but keep taste.
- Use skinless chicken thighs, instead of neck bones.

Oils/Butter
- Use cooking oil spray to lower fat and calories.
- Use a small amount of vegetable oil, instead of lard, butter, or other fats that are hard at room temperature.
- In general, diet margarines are not well suited for baking—instead, to cut saturated fat, use regular soft margarine made with vegetable oil.
- Choose margarine that lists liquid vegetable oil as the first ingredient on the food label and is low in saturated fat and low in or free of *trans* fat.

BOX 22 *(continued)*

Eggs
- In baking or cooking, use three egg whites and one egg yolk instead of two whole eggs, or two egg whites or ¼ cup of egg substitute instead of one whole egg.

Meats and Poultry
- Choose a lean cut of meat and remove any visible fat.
- Remove skin from chicken and other poultry before cooking.
- Try replacing beef with turkey in many recipes.

Sandwiches and Salads
- In salads and sandwiches, use fat-free or low-fat dressing, yogurt, or mayonnaise, instead of regular versions.
- To make a salad dressing, use equal parts water and vinegar, and half as much oil.
- Garnish salads with fruits and vegetables.

Soups and Stews
- Remove fat from homemade broths, soups, and stews by preparing them ahead and chilling them. Before reheating the dish, lift off the hardened fat that formed at the surface. If you don't have time to chill the dish, float a few ice cubes on the surface of the warm liquid to harden the fat. Then remove and discard the fat.
- Use cooking spray, water, or stock to sauté onion for flavoring stews, soups, and sauces.

Breads
- To make muffins, quick breads, and biscuits, use no more than 1–2 tablespoons of fat for each cup of flour.
- When making muffins or quick breads, use three ripe, very well-mashed bananas, instead of ½ cup butter or oil. Or substitute a cup of applesauce for a cup of butter, margarine, oil, or shortening—you'll get less saturated fat and fewer calories.

Desserts
- To make a pie crust, use only ½ cup margarine for every 2 cups of flour.
- For chocolate desserts, use 3 tablespoons of cocoa, instead of 1 ounce of baking chocolate. If fat is needed to replace that in chocolate, add 1 tablespoon or less of vegetable oil.
- To make cakes and soft-drop cookies, use no more than 2 tablespoons of fat for each cup of flour.

BOX 23

Eating Right When Eating Out

You can eat out without falling off the TLC diet, whether at a restaurant or a social event. When in a restaurant, don't hesitate to make special requests. Restaurants are used to such orders. At a social event, choose carefully but enjoy fully. Here are the tips:

At restaurants

- Choose entrees, potatoes, and vegetables prepared without sauces, cheese, or butter—or ask for sauces to be put on the side.
- Eat a small portion of meat—fill up on vegetables.
- Avoid vegetable and salad toppings, such as chopped eggs, crumbled bacon, and cheese—or tell the waiter you don't want these items in the dish.
- Ask for soft margarine instead of butter—and use it sparingly.
- Select foods which are steamed, garden fresh, broiled, baked, roasted, poached, and lightly sautéed or stir fried.
- At Chinese restaurants, look for items that are steamed, jum (poached), kow (roasted), or shu (barbecued). Ask for steamed rice and no MSG.
- At Italian restaurants, look for red sauces, primavera (no cream), piccata (lemon), sun-dried tomatoes, crushed tomatoes, lightly sautéed, or grilled.
- At Mexican restaurants, look for spicy chicken, rice and black beans, salsa or picante, or soft corn tortillas.
- If you order pizza, try a vegetable topping, instead of meat or extra cheese—or, ask for half the usual amount of cheese.
- At fast food restaurants, order salads, grilled chicken sandwiches with no breading, regular-size hamburgers, or roast beef sandwiches.

At social events

- If it's a buffet, look at all the offerings before you start filling your plate—and select mostly low-fat items. Take smaller servings of higher fat foods.
- At potluck dinners, bring a low-fat dish—that way, you'll have at least one food you're sure you can eat.
- At parties, sit away from the food table to avoid temptation.
- Tell hosts that you're on a cholesterol-lowering diet and ask if low-fat foods can be included on the menu.

BOX 24

Benefits of Regular Physical Activity

Regular physical activity is good for you in many ways in addition to helping you raise HDL and lower LDL:

- Physical activity is good for your heart.
- Your weight is much easier to control when you are active.
- Physical activity can boost your ability to make other improvements in lifestyle such as diet changes.
- You'll feel and look better when you're physically active.
- You'll feel more confident when you are active.
- Physical activity is a great way to burn off steam and stress and helps you beat the blues.
- You'll have more energy.
- You can share physical activities with friends and family.
- Physical activity can be lots of fun.

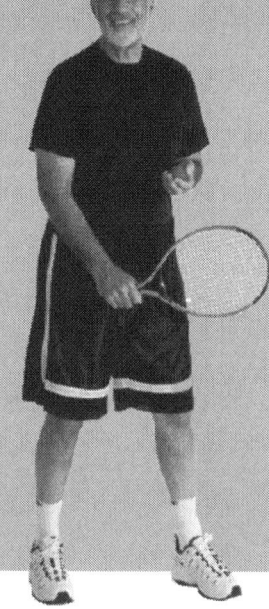

should check with your doctor before starting your physical activity program.

Unless your doctor tells you otherwise, try to get at least 30 minutes of a moderate-intensity activity such as brisk walking on most, and preferably all, days of the week. You can do the activity all at once or break it up into shorter periods of at least 10 minutes each. Moderate-intensity activities include playing golf (walking the course, instead of riding in a cart), dancing, bowling, bicycling (5 miles in 30 minutes), as well as gardening and house cleaning. More intense activities include jogging, swimming, doing aerobics, or playing basketball, football, soccer, racquetball, or tennis. Box 25 offers tips on how to become physically active. Box 26 shows how many calories you burn with different activities. Box 27 (page 46) gives guidelines on how to avoid injury as you become physically active.

Maintaining a Healthy Weight.

Being overweight or obese increases your chances for having high triglycerides, a low HDL, and a high LDL. You're also more likely to develop high blood pressure, diabetes, heart disease, some cancers, and other serious health problems. If you have excess weight around your waist, you're more likely to develop the metabolic syndrome (see pages 70–72).

Losing your extra weight reduces these risks and improves your cholesterol and triglyceride levels.

If you are overweight and have a high cholesterol, you'll need to get your LDL and your weight under control by changing your diet and increasing your physical activity. At the start of the TLC program, your main focus will be on lowering LDL toward the goal level (see pages 6–12) by making changes such as reducing saturated fat and calories and increasing fiber, which could also help you lose weight.

BOX 25

Getting Active

You don't have to train like a marathon runner to get the benefits of physical activity. If you're new to physical activity, start slowly and build gradually. Here's how:

Beginning Activity

Try to increase standing activities and special chores such as painting a room, pushing a stroller or wheelchair, doing yard work, ironing, cooking, or playing a musical instrument.

Light Activity

As you become more able to do a physical activity, try something light, such as walking slowly (a 24-minute mile),* garage work, carpentry, house cleaning, child care, golf, sailing, or recreational table tennis.

Moderate-Intensity Activity

Now you can try walking a 15-minute mile,* weeding and hoeing a garden, cycling, skiing, playing tennis, or dancing.

High-Intensity Activity

You're set to try walking a 10-minute mile,* walking uphill with a load, playing basketball or soccer/kick ball, or climbing.

*If you are walking for physical activity, use a pedometer to keep track of how many steps you take a day, and gradually increase the number of steps.

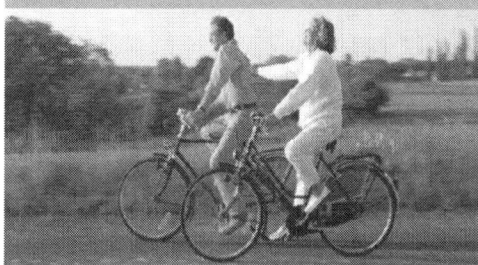

BOX 26

A Handy Guide to Calories Burned in Common Activities

Activity	Calories Burned Per 30 Minutes*
Walking (leisurely), 2 miles per hour	85
Walking (brisk), 4 miles per hour	170
Gardening	135
Raking leaves	145
Dancing	190
Bicycling (leisurely), 10 miles per hour	205
Swimming laps, medium level	240
Jogging, 5 miles per hour	275

For a healthy 150-pound person. A lighter person burns fewer calories; a heavier person burns more.

Each of these activities burns approximately 150 calories:

Example of Moderate Amounts of Physical Activity

Common Chores	Sports Activities	
Washing and waxing a car for 45–60 minutes	Playing volleyball for 45–60 minutes	↑ Less Vigorous, More Time
Washing windows or floors for 45–60 minutes	Playing touch football for 45 minutes	
Gardening for 30–45 minutes	Walking 1½ miles in 35 minutes (20 minutes/mile)	
Wheeling self in wheelchair 30–40 minutes	Basketball (shooting baskets) for 30 minutes	
Pushing a stroller 1½ miles in 30 minutes	Bicycling 5 miles in 30 minutes	
Raking leaves for 30 minutes	Dancing fast (social) for 30 minutes	
Shoveling snow for 15 minutes	Walking 2 miles in 30 minutes (15 minutes/mile)	
Stair walking for 15 minutes	Water aerobics for 30 minutes	
	Swimming laps for 20 minutes	
	Basketball (playing game) for 15–20 minutes	
	Bicycling 4 miles in 15 minutes	
	Jumping rope for 15 minutes	
	Running 1½ miles in 15 minutes (10 minutes/mile)	↓ More Vigorous, Less Time

BOX 27

Safe Moves

Here are some guidelines to keep in mind as you become physically active—they'll help you avoid injury:

- **Go slow.** Before each activity session, allow a 5-minute period of slow movement to give your muscles a chance to warm up. At the end of your activity, take another 5 minutes to cool down with a slower, less energetic pace.
- **Listen to your body.** A certain amount of stiffness is normal at first. But if you hurt a joint or pull a muscle, stop the activity for several days to avoid more serious injury. Rest and over-the-counter painkillers can heal most minor muscle and joint problems.
- **Check the weather report.** Dress appropriately for hot, humid days and for cold days. In all weather, drink lots of water before, during, and after physical activity.
- **Pay attention to warning signals.** While physical activity can strengthen your heart, some types of activity may worsen existing heart problems. Warning signals include sudden dizziness, cold sweat, paleness, fainting, or pain or pressure in your upper body just after doing a physical activity. If you notice any of these signs, stop and call 9-1-1 at once.
- **Use caution.** If you're concerned about the safety of your surroundings, pair up with a buddy for outdoor activities. This is a good family activity too. Walk, bike, or jog during daylight hours—or try a walk at the mall.
- **Keep at it.** Unless you have to stop your activity for a health reason, stick with it. If you feel like giving up because you think you're not going as fast or as far as you should, set smaller, short-term goals. If you become bored, try doing a different activity, or do an activity with a friend. Switching activities is called "cross training." If you always walk on a treadmill, try a bicycle instead. If you're tired of aerobic videos, sign up for a boxing class. Plan your week so you switch back and forth.

After about 2–3 months of TLC, if you are still overweight, you may need to focus additional attention on losing weight as you approach your LDL goal, especially if you have the metabolic syndrome (see Box 8 on page 17).

Finding out if you need to lose weight involves a two-step process: First, your doctor may already have checked your body mass index, or BMI, which relates your weight to your height. The table in Box 28 gives BMIs for various heights and weights. A BMI of 18.5–24.9 indicates a normal weight; a BMI of 25–29.9 is overweight; while a BMI of 30 or higher is obese.

Second, your doctor may have taken your waist measurement. A waist measurement of 35 inches or more for women or 40 inches or more for men is one of the factors involved in the metabolic syndrome (see pages 70–72). It also indicates an increased risk of obesity-related conditions, such as heart disease.

Check with your doctor and find out what a healthy weight is for you. If you need to lose pounds, do so gradually—a reasonable and safe weight loss is 1 to 2 pounds a week. You don't have to reach your ideal weight to reap health benefits. If you are overweight, losing even 10 percent of your current weight lowers your risk for heart disease and other health problems.

Box 29 offers pointers on things you can do to help you lose weight. Follow the TLC diet, watch your calorie intake, and increase your physical activity. The TLC diet is low in saturated fat and cholesterol—which fights heart disease—and calls for only enough calories for you to reach or maintain a healthy weight. If you need to lose weight, you'll have to take in fewer calories than you burn—this includes calories used by the body in normal functions and in physical activities. To lose 1 pound a week, you need to eat 500 fewer calories a day than you use up. In general, eating plans containing 1,000–1,200 calories will help most women lose weight safely, while eating plans with 1,200–1,600 calories a day are suitable for men. Boxes 30 and 31 offer tips on how to reduce your calorie intake. If you need to lose weight, be aware that low fat and low calorie are not the same (see Box 32 page 53). This confusion may lead you to overeat when you eat low-fat because you may think you're getting a calorie-free ride. Unfortunately, there are no such rides. To be sure you avoid this error, use the food label to compare products' calorie totals.

BOX 28

Find Your BMI

Find your height in the left-hand column and your weight* in one of the columns to the right. The number at the top of that column will be your BMI.

BODY MASS INDEX

	21	22	23	24	25	26	27	28	29	30	31
4'10"	100	105	110	115	119	124	129	134	138	143	148
5'0"	107	112	118	123	128	133	138	143	148	153	158
5'1"	111	116	122	127	132	137	143	148	153	158	164
5'3"	118	124	130	135	141	146	152	158	163	169	175
5'5"	126	132	138	144	150	156	162	168	174	180	186
5'7"	134	140	146	153	159	166	172	178	185	191	198
5'9"	142	149	155	162	169	176	182	189	196	203	209
5'11"	150	157	165	172	179	186	193	200	208	215	222
6'1"	159	166	174	182	189	197	204	212	219	227	235
6'3"	168	176	184	192	200	208	216	224	232	240	248

Weight is measured with underwear but not shoes.

What Does Your BMI Mean?

Categories:

Normal weight: BMI = 18.5–24.9.

Overweight: BMI = 25–29.9.

Obese: BMI = 30 or greater.

Source: Clinical Guidelines on the Identification, Evaluation, and Treatment of Overweight and Obesity in Adults: The Evidence Report; National Heart, Lung, and Blood Institute, in cooperation with the National Institute of Diabetes and Digestive and Kidney Diseases; National Institutes of Health; NIH Publication 98-4083; June 1998.

BOX 29

Losing Weight—and Gaining Heart Health

Losing weight is important for lowering your LDL and for improving your overall good health. Even a small weight loss helps protect your heart.

There are no quick fixes for losing weight. You need to change your lifestyle—follow the TLC diet, reduce calories, and become physically active. Your goal is not just to lose extra weight but to keep it off.

Losing weight isn't easy—in fact, it's a challenge. Here are some pointers to help you reach and keep your weight goal—for more tips, check the advice on pages 73–77 about how to change behaviors:

- **Change the way you eat.** You can eat less without feeling deprived. Here are three ways to decrease calories without decreasing satisfaction:
    1. Studies show that it takes at least 15 minutes for your brain to get the message that you've eaten. So slow down. Take time to savor your food.
    2. Eat more vegetables and fruits—they give a sense of fullness without adding a lot of calories.
    3. Use smaller plates. Your servings will seem bigger.

- **Beware of eating triggers.** You probably have come to associate certain behaviors with eating. For example, you may reach for the potato chips when you watch TV. Or you may overeat when dining with friends. These behaviors trigger your eating. Try to change the behavior in order to avoid the eating. Watch TV while riding an exercise bike. Do an activity with friends other than dining out—go to a museum, for example.

- **Don't skip meals.** Skipping or delaying meals can make you very hungry—causing you to overeat.

BOX 30

How To Lower Calories on TLC

When it comes to weight loss, there's only one equation that works: Eat less and be more physically active. The tips below will help you scale back your calorie intake—also check out the cooking methods in Box 22 on pages 39–40.

- Drink at least eight 8-ounce glasses of water or other noncaloric beverages each day to help you feel full.
- If you get hungry, eat some fresh or steamed vegetables.
- Start a meal with a broth-based soup.
- Choose very lean forms of protein—they are low in calories and fat. For example:
1 ounce of turkey breast or chicken with the skin removed, 1 ounce of fish fillets (flounder, sole, scrod, cod, haddock, or halibut), 1 ounce of canned tuna in water, 3/4 cup of fat-free or low-fat cottage cheese, 2 egg whites or 1/4 cup of egg substitute, 1 ounce of fat-free cheese, and 1/2 cup of cooked beans (black beans, kidney beans, chickpeas, or lentils).
- Have lean beef, veal, lamb, or pork only 1–2 times a week.
- Go for fruits—they have less than 100 calories per serving. For example: 1 small apple, banana, orange, or nectarine; 1 medium fresh peach; 1 kiwi; 1/2 grapefruit; 1/2 mango; 1 cup of fresh berries (strawberries, raspberries, or blueberries); 1 cup of fresh melon cubes; 1/8 of a honeydew melon; 4 ounces of unsweetened juice; 4 teaspoons jelly or jam.
- Use reduced calorie or "lite" bread—2 slices are about 80 calories, while regular breads have about twice as many calories.
- Shave calories when preparing and serving foods. Examples are: Try a little salsa on a baked potato instead of butter; use reduced fat Italian dressing on salads instead of the regular version.

BOX 31

Choose the Foods That Help You Lose

Learn to pick lower calorie versions of foods. But to lose weight and stay healthy, don't forget to get enough vitamins and minerals. Some foods provide most of their calories from sugar or fat and give few, if any, vitamins and minerals. Also, women in particular should be sure to have enough calcium—1,000–1,500 milligrams a day (through food or supplements). So choose foods wisely and lose weight well.

Here are some examples:

Instead of	Replace With
Cheddar, swiss, jack cheese	Reduced-calorie cheese, low-calorie processed cheeses
American cheese	Fat-free American cheese or other types of fat-free cheeses
Ramen noodles	Rice or noodles (such as spaghetti, macaroni)
Pasta with white sauce (alfredo)	Pasta with red sauce (marinara)
Pasta with cheese sauce	Pasta with vegetables (primavera)
Granola	Bran flakes, crispy rice cereals Cooked grits or oatmeal Whole grains (such as couscous, barley, bulgur) Reduced-fat granola
Creamed soups	Canned broth-based soups
Gravy (homemade with fat and/or milk)	Gravy mixes made with water or homemade with the fat skimmed off and fat-free milk included
Avocado on sandwiches	Cucumber slices or lettuce leaves
Guacamole dip or refried beans with lard	Salsa

BOX 31 *(continued)*

Instead of	Replace With
Cold cuts or lunch meats (such as bologna, salami, liverwurst)	Low-fat cold cuts (95-97% fat-free lunch meats, low-fat processed meats)
Hot dogs (regular)	Lower fat hot dogs
Bacon or sausage	Canadian bacon or lean ham
Regular ground beef	Extra lean ground beef (such as ground round or ground turkey)
Beef (chuck, rib, brisket)	Beef (round, loin and trimmed of external fat)
Croissants, brioches	Hard French rolls or soft "brown 'n serve" rolls
Donuts, sweet rolls, muffins, scones, or pastries	English muffins, bagels, reduced-fat or fat-free, muffins or scones
Party crackers	Low-fat crackers, saltine or soda crackers (lower in sodium)
Cake (pound, chocolate, yellow)	Cake (angel food, white, gingerbread)
Cookies	Reduced-fat or fat-free, low-calorie cookies (graham crackers, ginger snaps, fig bars—compare calorie levels)
Nuts	Air-popped or light microwave popcorn, fruits, vegetables
Ice cream	Sorbet, sherbet, fat-free frozen yogurt, frozen fruit, or chocolate pudding bars
Custard or puddings made with whole milk	Puddings made with skim milk

Choose the Foods That Help You Lose

BOX 32

When It Comes to Weight Loss—Fat Matters But Calories Count

Reducing the amount of saturated fat in your diet is important to lower a high LDL-cholesterol level. Eating less total fat can help reduce saturated fat, and also can help limit your overall calorie intake, since many high-fat foods are also high in calories. But eating fat-free or reduced-fat foods isn't always the answer.

A calorie is a calorie, whatever its source. Whether it comes from fat, or carbohydrates, or protein, it's still a calorie. So eating reduced-fat or fat-free foods won't necessarily lower your calorie intake. Some of these foods have as much or more calories than the regular versions. Further, you may be tempted to eat more of them because you think they're healthy. But if you eat twice as many fat-free cookies because you think they're healthy, you'll wind up taking in more calories. For example, 2 tablespoons of reduced-fat peanut butter have 187 calories—the same amount of regular peanut butter has 191 calories. So the reduced-fat version will cost you virtually the same number of calories. Similarly, half a cup of nonfat vanilla frozen yogurt has 100 calories—the same amount of regular whole milk vanilla frozen yogurt has 104 calories. If you're trying to lose weight, be sure you count calories.

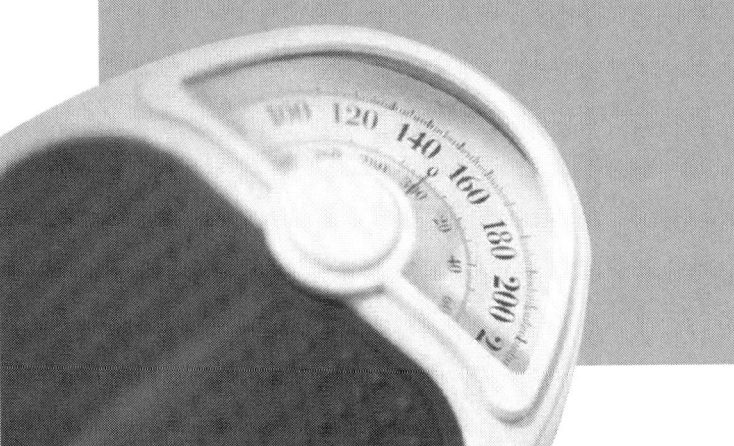

Another thing to keep an eye on is portion size. Studies show that portion sizes at restaurants and at home have gotten bigger in the past couple of decades. And most people eat what's on their plate. But portion size is not the same as serving size. A portion is the amount of a food you choose to eat at one sitting. A serving is a measure used to describe the amount of food recommended from each food group, and the size of a serving is shown on the Nutrition Facts label on the food package. Be sure to read the food label to learn how many servings are in a product—some items may appear to be sold as single portions but actually have more than one serving. See Box 33 for a guide to serving sizes. One trick to shrink your portion size at home is to use smaller plates. In a restaurant, try sharing the meal or taking part of it home.

You may want to talk with your doctor about getting help to lose weight. Various resources are available, including dietitians, who can help you better plan meals, and organized weight loss programs. Box 34 on page 56 offers tips on how to choose a weight loss program.

Sample Menus for TLC

Now that you have learned the basics of the TLC Program—the TLC diet, physical activity, and weight management—let's get down to the nitty gritty of what to eat for a whole day's meals. Sample menus to get you started eating the TLC way are shown on pages 58–69. There are four kinds of menus: for traditional American-style, Southern-style, Mexican American-style, and Asian American-style foods. The men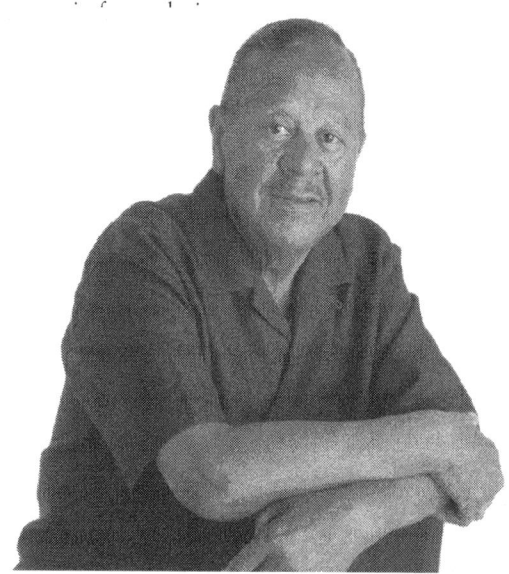
levels: 2,500 and 1,8(
women, respectively,
their LDL cholesterol
lose weight, and 1,60
to help also with weig
your doctor about th(
level that is right for

BOX 33

A Guide to Serving Sizes

The chart below shows what the serving sizes are for different food groups. Also, check out the Portion Distortion Interactive Quiz at: http://hin.nhlbi.nih.gov/portion/.

Serving Sizes for Food Groups

1 Serving Looks Like...

Grains
- 1 cup of cereal flakes = fist
- 1 pancake = compact disc
- ½ cup of cooked rice, pasta, or potato = ½ baseball
- 1 slice of bread = cassette tape
- 1 piece of cornbread = bar of soap

1 Serving Looks Like...

Fruit and Vegetables
- 1 med fruit = baseball
- ½ cup of fresh fruit = ½ baseball
- ¼ cup of raisins = large egg
- 1 cup of salad greens = baseball
- 1 baked potato = fist

1 Serving Looks Like...

Milk
- 1½ oz cheese = 4 stacked dice or 2 cheese slices
- ½ cup of ice cream = ½ baseball

Fats/Oils
- 1 tsp margarine or spreads = 1 die

1 Serving Looks Like...

Lean Meat and Beans
- 3 oz meat, fish, and poultry = deck of cards
- 3 oz grilled/baked fish = checkbook
- 2 Tbsp peanut butter = ping pong ball

BOX 34

Choosing a Weight Loss Program

Some people lose weight on their own, but others prefer the support given by a structured weight loss program. If you're considering joining such a program, be sure you know its total cost and its history of success—what percentage of those who start the program complete it; what percentage have problems or side effects (and what those are); and the average weight loss among those who finish the program. Look for a program that:

- Helps you lose weight slowly. Lose about 1 to 2 pounds a week. Quick fixes may be appealing but they do not last.

- Incorporates the TLC diet and offers flexible food choices. The program also should make allowances for your food likes and dislikes, as well as your lifestyle.

- Offers counseling to help you change your eating habits. It should help teach you how to change your eating and lifestyle habits—for the rest of your life. For instance, does the program give you tips on how to cope with times when you slip back into old habits?

- Gives you long-term strategies to keep the weight off. Such strategies may include having you set goals for types of physical activity, keep a weight and physical activity diary, vary types of or locations for physical activity, create a support system of friends/family/coworkers, or develop workout partners.

- Can help you keep weight off. Pick a program that will enhance your personal skills and give you techniques to keep you from regaining the lost weight.

- Has a professional staff. Qualified professionals who can help you lose weight safely and effectively include nutritionists and registered dietitians, doctors, nurses, psychologists, and exercise physiologists.

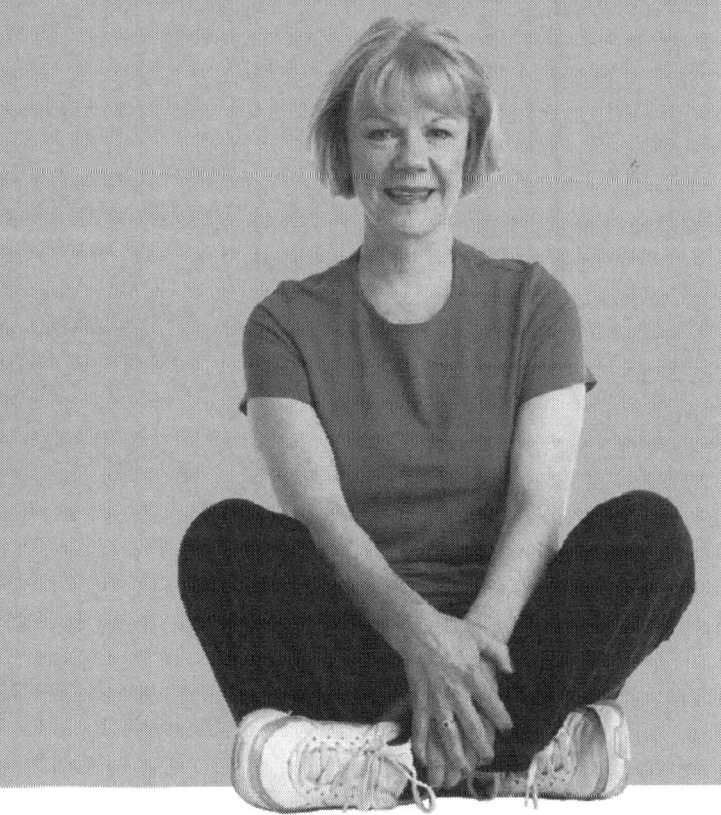

TLC Sample Menu
Traditional American Cuisine
2,500 Calories

Breakfast
Oatmeal (1 cup)
  Fat-free milk (1 cup)
  Raisins (¼ cup)
English muffin (1 medium)
  Soft margarine (2 tsp)
  Jelly (1 Tbsp)
Honeydew melon (1 cup)
Orange juice, calcium fortified (1 cup)
Coffee (1 cup) with fat-free milk (2 Tbsp)

Lunch
Roast beef sandwich
  Whole-wheat bun (1 medium)
  Roast beef, lean (2 oz)
  Swiss cheese, low fat (1 oz slice)
  Romaine lettuce (2 leaves)
  Tomato (2 medium slices)
  Mustard (2 tsp)
Pasta salad (1 cup)
  Pasta noodles (¾ cup)
  Mixed vegetables (¼ cup)
  Olive oil (2 tsp)
Apple (1 medium)
Iced tea, unsweetened (1 cup)

Dinner
Orange roughy (3 oz) cooked with olive oil (2 tsp)
Parmesan cheese (1 Tbsp)
Rice* (1½ cup)
Corn kernels (½ cup)
  Soft margarine (1 tsp)
Broccoli (½ cup)
  Soft margarine (1 tsp)
Roll (1 small)
  Soft margarine (1 tsp)
Strawberries (1 cup) topped with low-fat frozen yogurt (½ cup)
Fat-free milk (1 cup)

Snack
Popcorn (2 cups) cooked with canola oil (1 Tbsp)
Peaches, canned in water (1 cup)
Water (1 cup)

Nutrient Analysis

Calories	2,523	Total fat, % calories	28
Cholesterol (mg)	139	Saturated fat, % calories	6
Fiber (g)	32	Monounsaturated fat, % calories	14
Soluble (g)	10	Polyunsaturated fat, % calories	6
Sodium (mg)	1,800		
Carbohydrates, % calories	57	Protein, % calories	17

*Higher Fat Alternative

Total fat, % calories	34

No salt is added in recipe preparation or as seasoning.

* For a higher fat alternative, substitute ⅓ cup of unsalted peanuts, chopped (to sprinkle on the frozen yogurt) for 1 cup of the rice.

TLC Sample Menu
Traditional American Cuisine
1,800 Calories

Breakfast
Oatmeal (1 cup)
   Fat-free milk (1 cup)
   Raisins (¼ cup)
Honeydew melon (1 cup)
Orange juice, calcium fortified
   (1 cup)
Coffee (1 cup) with fat-free milk
   (2 Tbsp)

Lunch
Roast beef sandwich
   Whole-wheat bun (1 medium)
   Roast beef, lean (2 oz)
   Swiss cheese, low fat (1 oz slice)
   Romaine lettuce (2 leaves)
   Tomato (2 medium slices)
   Mustard (2 tsp)
Pasta salad (½ cup)
   Pasta noodles (¼ cup)
   Mixed vegetables (¼ cup)
   Olive oil (1 tsp)
Apple (1 medium)
Iced tea, unsweetened (1 cup)

Dinner
Orange roughy (2 oz) cooked with
   olive oil (2 tsp)
   Parmesan cheese (1 Tbsp)
Rice* (1 cup)
   Soft margarine (1 tsp)
Broccoli (½ cup)
   Soft margarine (1 tsp)
Strawberries (1 cup) topped with
   low-fat frozen yogurt (½ cup)
Water (1 cup)

Snack
Popcorn (2 cups) cooked with
   canola oil (1 Tbsp)
Peaches, canned in water (1 cup)
Water (1 cup)

Nutrient Analysis

Calories	1,795	Total fat, % calories	27
Cholesterol (mg)	115	Saturated fat, % calories	6
Fiber (g)	28	Monounsaturated fat, % calories	14
Soluble (g)	9	Polyunsaturated fat, % calories	6
Sodium (mg)	1,128		
Carbohydrates, % calories	57	Protein, % calories	19

*Higher Fat Alternative

Total fat, % calories	33

No salt is added in recipe preparation or as seasoning.

* *For a higher fat alternative, substitute 2 Tbsp of unsalted peanuts, chopped (to sprinkle on the frozen yogurt) for ½ cup of the rice.*

TLC Sample Menu
Southern Cuisine
2,500 Calories

Breakfast
Bran cereal (3/4 cup)
Banana (1 medium)
Fat-free milk (1 cup)
Biscuit, made with canola oil (1 medium)
Jelly (1 Tbsp)
Soft margarine (2 tsp)
Honeydew melon (1 cup)
Orange juice, calcium fortified (1 cup)
Coffee (1 cup) with fat-free milk (2 Tbsp)

Lunch
Chicken breast (3 oz), sautéed with canola oil (2 tsp)
Collard greens (1/2 cup)
Chicken broth, low sodium (1 Tbsp)
Black-eyed peas (1/2 cup)
Corn on the cob* (1 medium)
Soft margarine (1 tsp)
Rice, cooked (1 cup)
Soft margarine (1 tsp)
Fruit cocktail, canned in water (1 cup)
Iced tea, unsweetened (1 cup)

Dinner
Catfish (3 oz) coated with flour and baked with canola oil (1/2 Tbsp)
Sweet potato (1 medium)
Soft margarine (2 tsp)
Spinach (1/2 cup)
Vegetable broth, low sodium (2 Tbsp)
Corn muffin (1 medium), made with fat-free milk and egg substitute
Soft margarine (1 tsp)
Watermelon (1 cup)
Iced tea, unsweetened (1 cup)

Snack
Bagel (1 medium)
Peanut butter, reduced fat, unsalted (1 Tbsp)
Fat-free milk (1 cup)

Nutrient Analysis

Calories	2,504	Total fat, % calories	30
Cholesterol (mg)	158	Saturated fat, % calories	5
Fiber (g)	52	Monounsaturated fat, % calories	13
Soluble (g)	10	Polyunsaturated fat, % calories	9
Sodium (mg)	2,146		
Carbohydrates, % calories	59	Protein, % calories	18

*Higher Fat Alternative

Total fat, % calories	34

No salt is added in recipe preparation or as seasoning.

* *For a higher fat alternative, substitute 1/4 cup of unsalted almond slices for the corn on the cob. Sprinkle the almonds on the rice.*

TLC Sample Menu
Southern Cuisine
1,800 Calories

Breakfast
Bran cereal (³/4 cup)
Banana (1 medium)
Fat-free milk (1 cup)
Biscuit, low sodium and made with canola oil (1 medium)
Jelly (1 Tbsp)
Soft margarine (1 tsp)
Honeydew melon (¹/2 cup)
Coffee (1 cup) with fat-free milk (2 Tbsp)

Lunch
Chicken breast (2 oz) cooked with canola oil (2 tsp)
Corn on the cob* (1 medium)
Soft margarine (1 tsp)
Collard greens (¹/2 cup)
Chicken broth, low sodium (1 Tbsp)
Rice, cooked (¹/2 cup)
Fruit cocktail, canned in water (1 cup)
Iced tea, unsweetened (1 cup)

Dinner
Catfish (3 oz), coated with flour and baked with canola oil (¹/2 Tbsp)
Sweet potato (1 medium)
Soft margarine (2 tsp)
Spinach (¹/2 cup)
Vegetable broth, low sodium (2 Tbsp)
Corn muffin (1 medium), made with fat-free milk and egg substitute
Soft margarine (1 tsp)
Watermelon (1 cup)
Iced tea, unsweetened (1 cup)

Snack
Graham crackers (4 large)
Peanut butter, reduced fat, unsalted (1 Tbsp)
Fat-free milk (¹/2 cup)

Nutrient Analysis

Calories	1,823	Total fat, % calories	30
Cholesterol (mg)	131	Saturated fat, % calories	5
Fiber (g)	43	Monounsaturated fat, % calories	14
Soluble (g)	8	Polyunsaturated fat, % calories	8
Sodium (mg)	1,676		
Carbohydrates, % calories	59	Protein, % calories	18

Higher Fat Alternative

Total fat, % calories	35

No salt is added in recipe preparation or as seasoning.

* For a higher fat alternative, substitute ¹/4 cup of unsalted almond slices for the corn on the cob. Sprinkle the almonds on the rice.

TLC Sample Menu
Mexican-American Cuisine
2,500 Calories

Breakfast
Bean Tortilla
  Corn tortilla (2 medium)
  Pinto beans* (1/2 cup)
  Onion (1/4 cup), tomato,
    chopped (1/4 cup)
  Jalapeno pepper (1 medium)
  Sauté with canola oil (1 tsp)
Papaya† (1 medium)
Orange Juice, calcium fortified (1 cup)
Coffee (1 cup) with fat-free milk
  (2 Tbsp)

Lunch
Stir-fried beef
  Sirloin steak (3 oz)
  Garlic, minced (1 tsp)
  Onion, chopped (1/4 cup)
  Tomato, chopped (1/4 cup)
  Potato, diced (1/4 cup)
  Salsa (1/4 cup)
  Olive oil (2 tsp)
Mexican rice
  Rice, cooked (1 cup)
  Onion, chopped (1/4 cup)
  Tomato, chopped (1/4 cup)
  Jalapeno pepper (1 medium)
  Carrots, diced (1/4 cup)
  Cilantro (2 Tbsp)
  Olive oil (1 Tbsp)
Mango (1 medium)
Blended fruit drink (1 cup)
  Fat-free milk (1 cup)

Lunch (continued)
  Mango, diced (1/4 cup)
  Banana, sliced (1/4 cup)
  Water (1/4 cup)

Dinner
Chicken fajita
  Corn tortilla (2 medium)
  Chicken breast, baked (3 oz)
  Onion, chopped (2 Tbsp)
  Green pepper, chopped (1/4 cup)
  Garlic, minced (1 tsp)
  Salsa (2 Tbsp)
  Canola oil (2 tsp)
Avocado salad
  Romaine lettuce (1 cup)
  Avocado slices, dark skin,
    California type (1 small)
  Tomato, sliced (1/4 cup)
  Onion, chopped (2 Tbsp)
  Sour cream, low fat (1 1/2 Tbsp)
Rice pudding with raisins (3/4 cup)
Water (1 cup)

Snack
Plain yogurt, fat free, no sugar
  added (1 cup)
  Mixed with peaches, canned in
    water (1/2 cup)
Water (1 cup)

Nutrient Analysis

Calories	2,535	Total fat, % calories	28
Cholesterol (mg)	158	Saturated fat, % calories	5
Fiber (g)	48	Monounsaturated fat, % calories	17
Soluble (g)	17	Polyunsaturated fat, % calories	5
Sodium (mg)	2,118		
Carbohydrates, % calories	58	Protein, % calories	17

*Higher Fat Alternative

Total fat, % calories	33

No salt is added in recipe preparation or as seasoning.

* For a higher fat alternative, cook beans with canola oil (1 Tbsp).
† If using higher fat alternative, reduce papaya serving to 1/2 medium fruit because canola oil adds extra calories.

TLC Sample Menu
Mexican-American Cuisine
1,800 Calories

Breakfast
Bean Tortilla
  Corn tortilla (1 medium)
  Pinto beans (¼ cup)
  Onion (2 Tbsp), tomato,
    chopped (2 Tbsp)
  Jalapeno pepper (1 medium)
    Sauté with canola oil (1 tsp)
Papaya* (1 medium)
Orange juice, calcium fortified
  (1 cup)
Coffee (1 cup) with fat-free milk
  (2 Tbsp)

Lunch
Stir-fried Beef
  Sirloin steak (2 oz)
  Garlic, minced (1 tsp)
  Onion, chopped (¼ cup)
  Tomato, chopped (¼ cup)
  Potato, diced† (¼ cup)
  Salsa (¼ cup)
  Olive oil (1½ tsp)
Mexican rice (½ cup)
  Rice, cooked (½ cup)
  Onion, chopped (2 Tbsp)
  Tomato, chopped (2 Tbsp)
  Jalapeno pepper (1 medium)
  Carrots, diced (2 Tbsp)
  Cilantro (1 Tbsp)
  Olive oil (2 tsp)
Mango (1 medium)

Lunch (continued)
  Blended fruit drink (1 cup)
    Fat free milk (1 cup)
    Mango, diced (¼ cup)
    Banana, sliced (¼ cup)
    Water (¼ cup)

Dinner
Chicken fajita
  Corn tortilla (1 medium)
  Chicken breast, baked (2 oz)
  Onion, chopped (2 Tbsp)
  Green pepper, chopped (2 Tbsp)
  Garlic, minced (1 tsp)
  Salsa (1½ Tbsp)
  Canola oil (1 tsp)
Avocado salad
  Romaine lettuce (1 cup)
  Avocado slices, dark skin,
    California type (½ small)
  Tomato, sliced (¼ cup)
  Onion, chopped (2 Tbsp)
  Sour cream, low-fat (1½ Tbsp)
Rice pudding with raisins (½ cup)
Water (1 cup)

Snack
Plain yogurt, fat-free, no sugar
  added (1 cup)
  Mixed with peaches, canned in
    water (½ cup)
Water (1 cup)

Nutrient Analysis

Calories	1,821	Total fat, % calories	26
Cholesterol (mg)	110	Saturated fat, % calories	4
Fiber (g)	35	Monounsaturated fat, % calories	15
Soluble (g)	13	Polyunsaturated fat, % calories	4
Sodium (mg)	1,739		
Carbohydrates, % calories	61	Protein, % calories	17

*Higher Fat Alternative

Total fat, % calories	34	No salt is added in recipe preparation or as seasoning.

* If using higher fat alternative, eliminate papaya because the peanuts add extra calories.
† For a higher fat alternative, substitute ½ cup of unsalted peanut halves for the potato.

TLC Sample Menu
Asian Cuisine
2,500 Calories

Breakfast
Scrambled egg whites (³/4 cup liquid egg substitute)
Cooked with fat-free cooking spray*
English muffin (1 whole)
Soft margarine (2 tsp)
Jam (1 Tbsp)
Strawberries (1 cup)
Orange juice, calcium fortified† (1 cup)
Coffee (1 cup) with fat-free milk (2 Tbsp)

Lunch
Tofu Vegetable stir-fry
Tofu (3 oz)
Mushrooms (¹/2 cup)
Onion (¹/4 cup)
Carrots (¹/2 cup)
Swiss chard (1 cup)
Garlic, minced (2 Tbsp)
Peanut oil (1 Tbsp)
Soy sauce, low sodium (2¹/2 tsp)
Rice, cooked (1 cup)
Vegetable egg roll, baked (1 medium)
Orange (1 medium)
Green Tea (1 cup)

Dinner
Beef stir-fry
Beef tenderloin (3 oz)
Soybeans, cooked (¹/4 cup)
Broccoli, cut in large pieces (¹/2 cup)
Carrots, sliced (¹/2 cup)
Peanut oil (1 Tbsp)
Soy sauce, low sodium (2 tsp)
Rice, cooked (1 cup)
Watermelon (1 cup)
Almond cookies (2 cookies)
Fat-free milk (1 cup)

Snack
Chinese noodles, soft (1 cup)
Peanut oil (2 tsp)
Banana (1 medium)
Green tea (1 cup)

Nutrient Analysis

Calories	2,519	Total fat, % calories	28
Cholesterol (mg)	108	Saturated fat, % calories	5
Fiber (g)	37	Monounsaturated fat, % calories	11
Soluble (g)	15	Polyunsaturated fat, % calories	9
Sodium (mg)	2,268		
Carbohydrates, % calories	57	Protein, % calories	18

*Higher Fat Alternative

Total fat, % calories	32

No salt is added in recipe preparation or as seasoning.

* For a higher fat alternative, cook egg whites with 1 Tbsp of canola oil.
† If using higher fat alternative, eliminate orange juice because canola oil adds calories.

TLC Sample Menu
Asian Cuisine
1,800 Calories

Breakfast
Scrambled egg whites (½ cup liquid egg substitute)
    Cooked with fat-free cooking spray*
English muffin (1 whole)
    Soft margarine (2 tsp)
    Jam (1 Tbsp)
Strawberries (1 cup)
Orange juice, calcium fortified† (1 cup)
Coffee (1 cup) with fat-free milk (2 Tbsp)

Lunch
Tofu Vegetable stir-fry
    Tofu (3 oz)
    Mushrooms (½ cup)
    Onion (¼ cup)
    Carrots (½ cup)
    Swiss chard (½ cup)
    Garlic, minced (2 Tbsp)
    Peanut oil (1 Tbsp)
    Soy sauce, low sodium (2½ tsp)
Rice, cooked (½ cup)
Orange (1 medium)
Green tea (1 cup)

Dinner
Beef stir-fry
    Beef tenderloin (3 oz)
    Soybeans, cooked (¼ cup)
    Broccoli, cut in large pieces (½ cup)
    Peanut oil (1 Tbsp)
    Soy sauce, low sodium (2 tsp)
Rice, cooked (½ cup)
Watermelon (1 cup)
Almond cookie (1 cookie)
Fat-free milk (1 cup)

Snack
Chinese noodles, soft (½ cup)
    Peanut oil (1 tsp)
Green tea (1 cup)

Nutrient Analysis

Calories	1,829	Total fat, % calories	28
Cholesterol (mg)	74	Saturated fat, % calories	6
Fiber (g)	26	Monounsaturated fat, % calories	11
Soluble (g)	10	Polyunsaturated fat, % calories	9
Sodium (mg)	1,766		
Carbohydrates, % calories	56	Protein, % calories	18

*Higher Fat Alternative

Total fat, % calories	33

No salt is added in recipe preparation or as seasoning.

* *For a higher fat alternative, cook egg whites with 1 Tbsp of canola oil.*
† *If using higher fat alternative, eliminate orange juice because canola oil adds extra calories.*

Traditional American Cuisine—Reduced Calories

	1,200 Calories	1,600 Calories
Breakfast		
Whole wheat bread	1 med slice	1 med slice
Jelly, regular	2 tsp	2 tsp
Cereal, shredded wheat	½ cup	1 cup
Milk, 1%	1 cup	1 cup
Orange juice	¾ cup	¾ cup
Coffee, regular	1 cup	1 cup with 1 oz of 1% milk
Lunch		
Roast beef sandwich:		
Whole wheat bread	2 med slices	2 med slices
Lean roast beef, unseasoned	2 oz	2 oz
American cheese, low fat and low sodium	—	1 slice, ¾ oz
Lettuce	1 leaf	1 leaf
Tomato	3 med slices	3 med slices
Mayonnaise, low calorie	1 tsp	2 tsp
Apple	1 med	1 med
Water	1 cup	1 cup
Dinner		
Salmon	2 oz edible	3 oz edible
Vegetable oil	1½ tsp	1½ tsp
Baked potato	¾ med	¾ med
Margarine	1 tsp	1 tsp
Green beans, seasoned, with margarine	½ cup	½ cup
Carrots, seasoned	½ cup	—
Carrots, seasoned, with margarine	—	½ cup
White dinner roll	1 small	1 med
Ice milk	—	½ cup
Iced tea, unsweetened	1 cup	1 cup
Water	2 cup	2 cup
Snack		
Popcorn	2½ cup	2½ cup
Margarine	¾ tsp	½ tsp

Calories	1,247	Calories	1,613
Total carbohydrate, % calories	58	Total carbohydrate, % calories	55
Total fat, % calories	26	Total fat, % calories	29
*Saturated fat, % calories	7	*Saturated fat, % calories	8
Sodium, mg	1,043	Sodium, mg	1,341
Cholesterol, mg	96	Cholesterol, mg	142
Protein, % calories	19	Protein, % calories	19

Note: Calories have been rounded. No salt added in recipe preparation or as seasoning.
*At these reduced calorie levels, the amount of saturated fat is low even if the percent of calories from saturated fat is slightly over 7 percent.

Southern Cuisine—Reduced Calories

	1,200 Calories	1,600 Calories
Breakfast		
Oatmeal, prepared with 1% milk, low fat	1/2 cup	1/2 cup
Milk 1%, low fat	1/2 cup	1/2 cup
English muffin	—	1 med
Cream cheese, light, 18% fat	—	1 Tbsp
Orange juice	1/2 cup	3/4 cup
Coffee	1 cup	1 cup
Milk 1%, low fat	1 oz	1 oz
Lunch		
Baked chicken, without skin	2 oz	2 oz
Vegetable oil	1/2 tsp	1 tsp
Salad:		
Lettuce	1/2 cup	1/2 cup
Tomato	1/2 cup	1/2 cup
Cucumber	1/2 cup	1/2 cup
Oil and vinegar dressing	1 tsp	2 tsp
White rice	1/4 cup	1/2 cup
Margarine, diet	1/2 tsp	1/2 tsp
Baking powder biscuit, prepared with vegetable oil	1/2 small	1 small
Margarine	1 tsp	1 tsp
Water	1 cup	1 cup
Dinner		
Lean roast beef	2 oz	3 oz
Onion	1/4 cup	1/4 cup
Beef gravy, water-based	1 Tbsp	1 Tbsp
Turnip greens	1/2 cup	1/2 cup
Margarine, diet	1/2 tsp	1/2 tsp
Sweet potato, baked	1 small	1 small
Margarine, diet	1/4 tsp	1/2 tsp
Ground cinnamon	1 tsp	1 tsp
Brown sugar	1 tsp	1 tsp
Corn bread prepared with margarine, diet	1/2 med slice	1/2 med slice
Honeydew melon	1/8 med	1/4 med
Iced tea, sweetened with sugar	1 cup	1 cup
Snack		
Saltine crackers, unsalted tops	4 crackers	4 crackers
Mozzarella cheese, part skim, low sodium	1 oz	1 oz

Calories	1,225	Calories		1,653
Total carbohydrate, % calories	50	Total carbohydrate, % calories		53
Total fat, % calories	31	Total fat, % calories		28
*Saturated fat, % calories	9	*Saturated fat, % calories		8
Sodium, mg	867	Sodium, mg		1,231
Cholesterol, mg	142	Cholesterol, mg		172
Protein, % calories	21	Protein, % calories		20

Note: Calories have been rounded. No salt added in recipe preparation or as seasoning.
* At these reduced calorie levels, the amount of saturated fat is low even if the percent of calories from saturated fat is slightly over 7 percent.

Mexican-American Cuisine—Reduced Calories

	1,200 Calories	1,600 Calories
Breakfast		
Cantaloupe	½ cup	1 cup
Farina, prepared with 1% low-fat milk	½ cup	½ cup
White bread	1 slice	1 slice
Margarine	1 tsp	1 tsp
Jelly	1 tsp	1 tsp
Orange juice	¾ cup	1½ cup
Milk, 1%, low fat	½ cup	½ cup
Lunch		
Beef enchilada:		
Tortilla, corn	2 tortillas	2 tortillas
Lean roast beef	2 oz	2½ oz
Vegetable oil	⅔ tsp	⅔ tsp
Onion	1 Tbsp	1 Tbsp
Tomato	4 Tbsp	4 Tbsp
Lettuce	½ cup	½ cup
Chili peppers	2 tsp	2 tsp
Refried beans, prepared with vegetable oil	¼ cup	¼ cup
Carrots	5 sticks	5 sticks
Celery	6 sticks	6 sticks
Milk, 1%, low fat	—	½ cup
Water	1 cup	—
Dinner		
Chicken taco:		
Tortilla, corn	1 tortilla	1 tortilla
Chicken breast, without skin	1 oz	2 oz
Vegetable oil	⅔ tsp	⅔ tsp
Cheddar cheese, low fat and low sodium	½ oz	1 oz
Guacamole	1 Tbsp	2 Tbsp
Salsa	1 Tbsp	1 Tbsp
Corn	½ cup	½ cup seasoned with ½ tsp margarine
Spanish rice without meat	½ cup	½ cup
Banana	½ large	1 large
Coffee	½ cup	1 cup
Milk, 1%, low fat	1 oz	1 oz

Calories	1,239	Calories	1,638
Total carbohydrate, % calories	58	Total carbohydrate, % calories	56
Total fat, % calories	26	Total fat, % calories	27
*Saturated fat, % calories	8	*Saturated fat, % calories	9
Sodium, mg	1,364	Sodium, mg	1,616
Cholesterol, mg	91	Cholesterol, mg	143
Protein, % calories	19	Protein, % calories	20

Note: Calories have been rounded. No salt added in recipe preparation or as seasoning.
* *At these reduced calorie levels, the amount of saturated fat is low even if the percent of calories from saturated fat is slightly over 7 percent.*

Asian-American Cuisine—Reduced Calories

	1,200 Calories	1,600 Calories
Breakfast		
Banana	1 small	1 small
Whole-wheat bread	1 slice	2 slices
Margarine	1 tsp	1 tsp
Orange juice	3/4 cup	3/4 cup
Milk 1%, low fat	3/4 cup	3/4 cup
Lunch		
Beef noodle soup, canned, low sodium	1/2 cup	1/2 cup
Chinese noodle and beef salad:		
Beef roast	2 oz	3 oz
Peanut oil	1 tsp	1 1/2 tsp
Soy sauce, low sodium	1 tsp	1 tsp
Carrots	1/2 cup	1/2 cup
Zucchini	1/2 cup	1/2 cup
Onion	1/4 cup	1/4 cup
Chinese noodles, soft-type	1/4 cup	1/4 cup
Apple	1 med	1 med
Tea, unsweetened	1 cup	1 cup
Dinner		
Pork stir-fry with vegetables:		
Pork cutlet	2 oz	2 oz
Peanut oil	1 tsp	1 tsp
Soy sauce, low sodium	1 tsp	1 tsp
Broccoli	1/2 cup	1/2 cup
Carrots	1/2 cup	1 cup
Mushrooms	1/2 cup	1/4 cup
Steamed white rice	1/2 cup	1 cup
Tea, unsweetened	1 cup	1 cup
Snack		
Almond cookies	—	2 cookies
Milk 1%, low fat	3/4 cup	3/4 cup

Calories	1,220	Calories	1,609
Total carbohydrate, % calories	55	Total carbohydrate, % calories	56
Total fat, % calories	27	Total fat, % calories	27
*Saturated fat, % calories	8	*Saturated fat, % calories	8
Sodium, mg	1,043	Sodium, mg	1,296
Cholesterol, mg	117	Cholesterol, mg	148
Protein, % calories	21	Protein, % calories	20

Note: Calories have been rounded. No salt added in recipe preparation or as seasoning.
* At these reduced calorie levels, the amount of saturated fat is low even if the percent of calories from saturated fat is slightly over 7 percent.

The Metabolic Syndrome— A Special Concern

If you have the metabolic syndrome, you have an increased risk for heart disease. The syndrome isn't a disease itself but a cluster of risk factors for heart disease and other disorders, such as diabetes. One risk factor alone increases your chance of developing heart disease—having a group of them boosts your risk more. This is true even though some of the factors in the metabolic syndrome may be at levels below those for full-fledged heart disease risk factors. In fact, research indicates that having the metabolic syndrome can raise your chance of developing heart disease and diabetes even if your LDL cholesterol isn't elevated.

Heredity can play a role in whether a person develops the metabolic syndrome, but its underlying causes are abdominal obesity—too large a waist—and physical inactivity. The metabolic syndrome also is related to a condition called "insulin resistance"—which can lead to diabetes. Insulin is a hormone that helps your body convert glucose (sugar) in the blood into energy. With insulin resistance, the body cannot properly use the insulin it produces. As more and more Americans have become obese in recent years, the problem of metabolic syndrome has become more widespread. Today about one-quarter of all adults in the United States have the metabolic syndrome.

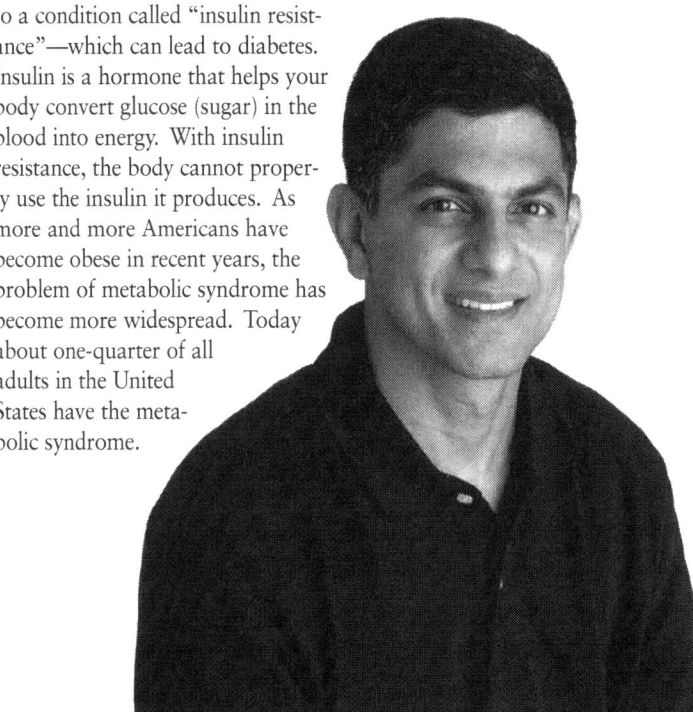

If you have three or more of the following factors, you have the metabolic syndrome:

- *Large waist measurement*—35 inches or more for women, 40 inches or more for men (this is also one of the measurements that determine if you need to lose weight)
- *Triglyceride* level of 150 mg/dL or higher
- *HDL cholesterol* of less than 50 mg/dL in women, less than 40 mg/dL in men
- *Blood pressure* of 130/85 mmHg or higher (either number counts as a raised blood pressure)
- *Fasting blood sugar* of 100 mg/dL or higher

If you have the metabolic syndrome, it is especially important for you to follow the TLC Program. Lifestyle changes are the main treatment for metabolic syndrome. TLC can help you reverse or reduce all of the metabolic syndrome's risk factors, which will reduce your risk of developing heart disease and diabetes.

Your first goal is to move toward getting your LDL under control. Then you'll focus on the risk factors of the metabolic syndrome. See Box 8 on page 17 for the steps of treatment.

The key parts of the TLC Program for treating the metabolic syndrome are:
- *Achieve a healthy weight* (see pages 43–57)
- *Become physically active* (see pages 37–46)
- *Follow the TLC diet* (see pages 19–41)

As was said earlier, the TLC diet calls for total fat to be 25–35 percent of the day's calories. Some experts recommend that people with the metabolic syndrome should aim for the higher end of this range—about 35 percent of calories from total fat. This is meant to keep carbohydrate consumption from being too high, which could further raise triglycerides and lower HDL. Other experts hold that, since weight loss is so important for treating the metabolic syndrome risk factors, a diet with less fat could be right for you if it helps you lose weight. Whichever diet you follow, remember to choose complex carbohydrates rather than simple sugars (see Box 20 on page 36). Some of the menus beginning on page 58 offer heart healthy options for having a higher fat intake on the TLC diet.

There are a couple of added points. First, if you have the metabolic syndrome and drink alcoholic beverages, it's doubly important to do so only in moderation. Drinking too many alcoholic beverages increases the risk for elevated triglycerides and high blood pressure. Further, alcoholic beverages add extra calories. So drinking too much also can add pounds. See page 30 for what "moderate drinking" means.

Second, the "don't smoke" advice that goes for everyone applies especially to you if you have the metabolic syndrome. Smoking tends to raise triglycerides and lower HDL. If you smoke, quitting can help reduce your triglyceride level and raise your HDL.

If lifestyle changes do not sufficiently control the metabolic syndrome risk factors, then drug therapy may be needed to manage one or more of them. For instance, you may need medication to treat high blood pressure, or elevated triglycerides and low HDL. Aspirin also may be prescribed to help prevent blood clots.

All of these actions will help reduce your risk for heart disease.

Learning To Live the TLC Way

Making lifestyle changes is never easy. But as you adopt the TLC Program, keep your key goal in mind: Living healthier and longer by lowering your cholesterol and other risk factors and reducing your risk for heart disease.

This section offers guidance on how to make the needed lifestyle changes. It also will describe how you can follow the TLC Program with your family and friends. In fact, your family and friends also can benefit from the program—it's never too early or too late to learn a heart healthy lifestyle. The key difference between your efforts and theirs is that yours must be more intense because you need to reverse a high cholesterol and/or other risk factors, not merely prevent them.

Also, remember to work closely with your doctor, dietitian, or other health care providers. Make them valuable members of your heart health improvement team. They can help you learn how to eat healthy, satisfying meals, find a weight loss program, or do physical activities safely and effectively.

Keeping Track of Your Changes

A good way to begin making changes is to *start a TLC diary*. This can be a diary of what you eat each day and other information, such as your physical activity and, if you need to lose pounds, your weight. Box 35 is a sample food and activity diary. You can copy it to record what you eat and what physical activity you do. But all it takes is a small notebook. Use the diary before you start on TLC to see what you need to change, and while on TLC to see how you are doing. Diaries help you keep on course and give you a boost by tracking your progress. A diary also can help your doctor, dietitian, or other health professional assess your progress.

If you are walking for physical activity, a pedometer is a good way to keep track of your progress. It tells you how many steps you've taken, so you can set a goal to increase your activity. Record your progress in your TLC diary.

BOX 35

Sample Food and Activity Diary

Use the sample diary below to record the foods you eat and the physical activity you do each day of the week.

Weekly Food and Activity Diary

	Monday	Tuesday	Wednesday
Breakfast			
Lunch			
Dinner			
Activity			

Notes
_____
_____
_____
_____

Thursday	Friday	Saturday	Sunday
		Week of:	

Be SMART When You Start

When you start making changes, try using the "SMART" approach. Whether it's reducing saturated fat, adding more fruits and vegetables to your meals, losing excess weight, or becoming more physically active—it's hard to change behaviors. But knowing how to approach a change helps make the change possible. And that's what the "SMART" approach does. It sets you up for success. Using this method, you set goals that are *Specific, Measured, Appropriate, Realistic,* and *Time-bound.*

Start by setting specific goals. For instance, if you need to increase your physical activity, saying you'll "do more now and then" is vague. It's hard to achieve a vague goal. But be sure the goal is also appropriate and realistic. For example, if you're not physically active, saying you'll walk 3 miles a day may be too much just yet. Instead, saying you'll walk an extra 2,000 steps a day gives you a specific aim—one that can be measured (using a pedometer), so you know when you succeed—and one that is also realistic. Nothing succeeds like success—so program yourself to be a winner.

Another key aspect of the SMART approach is to use those realistic, smaller steps to lead you toward your larger goal. For instance, if you're trying to switch from whole milk to fat-free milk, start by drinking 2-percent milk. Then, when you've achieved that change, move to 1-percent milk, and finally to fat-free milk. With this approach, you should stay motivated to make the entire journey.

Reward Yourself

Be sure to reward yourself for the progress you've made on TLC—but not with food. As you start a new goal, offer yourself a promise such as, "If I reach my goal this (day, week, month), I will treat myself to a well deserved (fill in a nonfood reward)." Think of something you want, such as a CD, a movie, or a massage. Or put down a deposit on a larger reward.

Making TLC a Family Affair
It's a good idea to talk about your plans for TLC with your spouse, family, or friends—whoever can provide support or needs to understand why you're changing your habits. They may even be able to help in concrete ways. For example, your spouse can help you plan heart healthier meals. In fact, you can follow the TLC program with your family.

You can follow the TLC diet without making separate meals for you and the rest of your family. The main difference between your diet and your family's is that yours has a lower intake of saturated fat and cholesterol than theirs. So you'll just eat less saturated fat and cholesterol than they do, or smaller portions.

How does this work at mealtimes? One approach is to use "add on's"—heart healthy sauces or foods that can be added to dishes so others can meet their nutrition goals while you keep to yours. Make salads and let everyone choose how much to add of nuts, seeds, raisins, or fruit. Put low-fat salad dressing and sauces on the side so others can have them.

Portion size is another way to share meals but remain on your TLC diet. Take less of the main course, such as meat, and more of the side dishes, such as vegetables.

At breakfast, top a whole grain English muffin with sugar-free preserves or jams, while others have a regular topping.

Family time should not mean only food. Physical activities also can be done with family or friends. Walking with your family or a friend can be fun—buddying-up can keep the activity from becoming dull. You'll also be sharing the heart health benefits.

Get your spouse to join a dance class with you. Invite your spouse or child or friend to play tennis with you regularly. Join a hiking or biking club. Start a softball team with family, neighbors, friends, or coworkers. Your family and friends may have other ideas too. Ask them and then get moving.

A Final Note

The TLC Program is a new way of living, not just a quick fix. So don't worry if you slip now and then. Don't let a slip keep you from reaching your health goals. Box 36 offers some advice about how to get back on track if you slip.

The biggest step is getting started. After that, take encouragement from your progress, and you'll reach your goal—a lifetime of heart health.

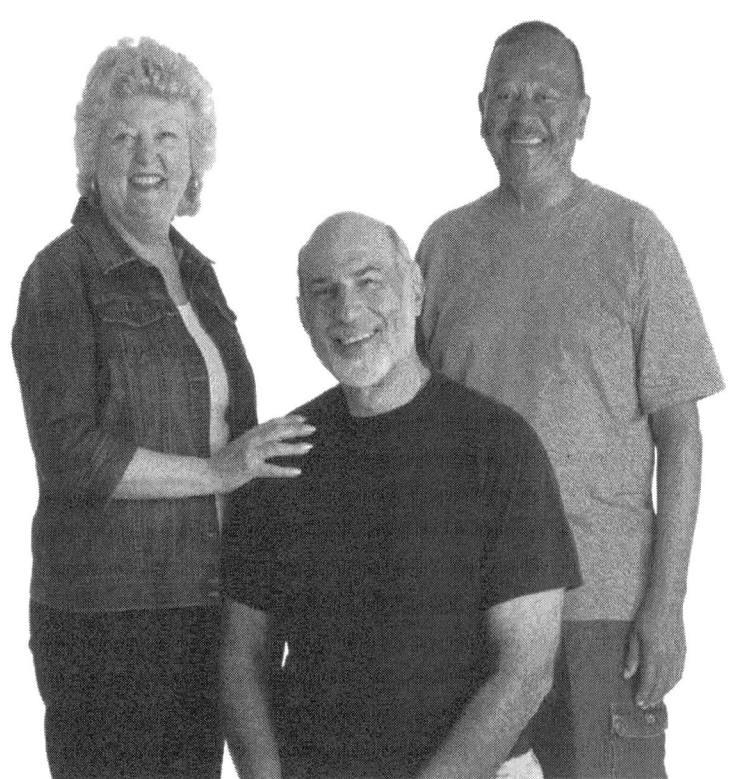

BOX 36

Getting Back on Track

You may slip from the TLC Program once in a while—not to worry. The important part is getting back on track. Here's how to do it:

- **Ask yourself why you got off track.** Did you eat the wrong foods at a party? Did you feel pressed for time and omit your physical activity? Find out what triggered your sidetrack and then get started again.
- **Don't worry about a slip.** Everyone does it—especially when learning something new. Remember that changing your lifestyle is a long-term process.
- **See if you tried to do too much at once.** Often, those starting a new lifestyle try to change too much at once. Slowly but surely is the best way to succeed.
- **Break the process down into small steps.** Remember, be a SMART planner (see page 76)—set reachable goals and keep your sights on the big prize of improved heart health.
- **Write it down.** Keep a food, physical activity, and weight diary. Record the what, when, where, how much—this can help you find the problem. You may want to put down such details as where you are and how you feel when you're eating the high saturated fat food or not doing your physical activity. It also can help you come up with solutions. For instance, if you find you keep eating a high saturated fat snack food while watching TV, you could keep a substitute healthier snack handy for those times.
- **Celebrate success.** Treat yourself to a reward—one that fits the TLC Program.

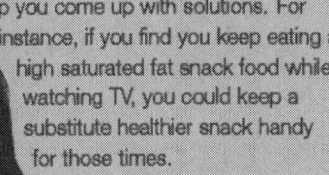

To Learn More

The National Heart, Lung, and Blood Institute (NHLBI) Health Information Center is a service of the NHLBI of the National Institutes of Health. The NHLBI Health Information Center provides information to health professionals, patients, and the public about the treatment, diagnosis, and prevention of heart, lung, and blood diseases and sleep disorders. For more information, contact:

NHLBI Health Information Center
P.O. Box 30105
Bethesda, MD 20824-0105
Phone: 301-592-8573
TTY: 240-629-3255
Fax: 301-592-8563
Web site: http://www.nhlbi.nih.gov

And check out these online resources:

Cholesterol
Live Healthier, Live Longer   www.nhlbi.nih.gov/chd

Weight
Aim for a Healthy Weight   www.nhlbi.nih.gov/subsites/index.htm
                                    - then click on Healthy Weight

Nutrition
U.S. Department of Agriculture   www.nutrition.gov

Physical Activity
The President's Council on   www.fitness.gov
Physical Fitness and Sports

High Blood Pressure
Your Guide to Lowering   www.nhlbi.nih.gov/hbp
High Blood Pressure

Smoking Cessation
Tobacco Information and   www.cdc.gov/tobacco/index.htm
Prevention Source—TIPS

Diabetes
National Diabetes Information   http://diabetes.niddk.nih.gov/
Clearinghouse

Discrimination Prohibited: Under provisions of applicable public laws enacted by Congress since 1964, no person in the United States shall, on the grounds of race, color, national origin, handicap, or age, be excluded from participation in, be denied the benefits of, or be subjected to discrimination under any program or activity (or, on the basis of sex, with respect to any education program or activity) receiving Federal financial assistance. In addition, Executive Order 11141 prohibits discrimination on the basis of age by contractors and subcontractors in the performance of Federal contracts, and Executive Order 11246 states that no federally funded contractor may discriminate against any employee or applicant for employment because of race, color, religion, sex, or national origin. Therefore, the National Heart, Lung, and Blood Institute must be operated in compliance with these laws and Executive Orders.

Made in the USA
Columbia, SC
01 February 2019